Healthy after 55

Now is the Time

Change Your Choices, Change Your Life

Julie Luedtke

Copyright © 2019 by Julie Luedtke.
All Rights Reserved.

No part of this publication may be reproduced, distributed, or transmitted in any form or by any means, including photocopying, recording, or other electronic or mechanical methods, or by any information storage and retrieval system without the prior written permission of the publisher, except in the case of very brief quotations embodied in critical reviews and certain other noncommercial uses permitted by copyright law.

DISCLAIMER

The information provided in this book is for educational purposes only. I am not a doctor and this is not meant to be taken as medical advice. The information provided in this guide is based on my experiences as well as my interpretation of the current research available.

The advice and tips given are meant for healthy adults only. Please consult your physician to ensure the tips given in the book are appropriate for your individual circumstances.

If you have any health issues or pre-existing conditions, please consult with your physical before implementing any of the information provided in this book.

This book is for informational purposes only and the author does not accept any responsibilities for any liabilities or damages, real or perceived, resulting from the use of this information.

I would like to dedicate this book to the following people:

My children, Kari, Bonnie and Scot. They encouraged me to write this book to share what I have learned so I could help more women regain and maintain their health. My children have encouraged me, kept me on track, and surrounded me with their love.

My accountability buddy, Ann, who kept me focused on the goal of writing this book. She gave great advice on content and editing, and we shared a lot of laughs along the way.

My fitness classes for women 55+ who encouraged me to share the knowledge that helped them regain their health and energy.

CONTENTS

Introduction 1

Chapter #1: Change Your Habits To Change Your Life. 7

Chapter #2: Right + Left = Balance 21

Chapter #3: Stir The Pot. 39

Chapter #4: Step It Up. 59

Chapter #5: Food Fight! 69

Chapter #6: Awareness. 86

Chapter #7: Choices. 99

Chapter #8: Restart 112

Chapter #9: Lifestyle Changes. 128

Chapter #10: What's Next 140

Chart Your Progress 149

About the Author. 151

One Last Thing 153

Introduction

Are you going to try a new diet program after your birthday?
Are you planning to join the local gym after the holidays?
Are you putting the needs of everyone else ahead of your own health?

IF YOU ANSWERED **YES** TO ANY OF THESE QUESTIONS, *now is the time to…*

- Focus on healthy eating instead of the latest diet

- Move more every day without stepping foot in a gym

- Make your health and wellness a priority

This realistic and motivating book will help you take practical, common sense steps to regain your health, and increase your strength and energy.

This book shows you how to take control of your health without an expensive gym membership or complicated food diary.

This step-by-step guide provides the information and motivation to help you feel better, increase your energy and boost your self-esteem.

As a woman over the age of 55, it's time for you to enjoy a vibrant, active lifestyle. You put the needs of others first for many years. *Now it is time to put **you** first!*

Here is a sample of what you'll discover in this book

- ★ Discover the real meaning of JOY

- ★ Learn the importance of movement

- ★ Reset how you think about food

- ★ Set realistic goals you can sustain over a life time

- ★ Launch your own personal healthy eating and movement plan

Your health is worth the effort. Take control of your life today.

Are you ready to take additional steps toward permanent lifestyle changes to a healthier, happier life?

If you didn't read the first book in this series, *"Healthy After 55 — Live Your Best Life,"* you can still begin your wellness journey right now with this book. This is a positive way to start your journey toward a healthy life.

Whether you are trying to regain your health and vitality, just beginning the journey of healthy living after 55, or looking for ways to maintain your health, this book is for you.

What makes this book different from all the other diet and exercise books on the market?

This book was created by someone who lives these steps every day.

I'm 74 and officially retired from corporate life. However, I continue to help other older adults live a vibrant, active life.

I am dedicated to helping you live your best life.

Many people search for ways to not only lead a healthier life, but a happier one as well.

Participants in my movement classes have been where you are right now. The difference? They took those first steps to gain control of their lives, and you can do the same thing.

As a certified personal trainer who has trained hundreds of older adults, I incorporate the steps in this book in classes I teach.

These steps have increased the health and happiness of participants. My students are the inspiration for this book. They are the focus group for what works and, just as importantly, what doesn't work.

My goal is to help **_you_** increase the *quality* of your life.

Quality of life becomes more important as we get older. You want to maintain your independence and live life with passion…no matter what the number is on your birth certificate.

I will take you through important steps to help you move more and change your eating habits.

Still Skeptical This Book Will Change Your Life?

A lady in one of my classes is a 66-year-old grandmother who struggled to get up off the floor by herself.

She came up to me with a big smile on her face after attending class for six weeks. She told me that by using the special way we practiced to get up off the floor, she could finally get up without any help after playing with her grandchildren.

That is just one example of how this book will change your life.

One Step At A Time…

This may seem overwhelming at first, but take it one step at a time. As you master each step, you will look forward to trying something new. There are plenty of pictures and charts to help you along the way.

Incorporating one step in your life is good, but integrating all of them together will help you achieve your goals.

Quality of life and your health are priceless! Once you begin the journey and see for yourself what you can accomplish, you will have the confidence to move forward with a happier, healthier outlook on life.

Are you ready to take this exciting step in your life's journey?

No more excuses.
LET'S GO!
Health is your first wealth!

NOTE: Whenever I work with an individual as a personal trainer, or in a class setting, I always confirm that the participants have checked with their health care professional before beginning any new program. I ask them to share with me what their health care professional told them regarding what they should do to increase their health and what they should avoid to prevent injury.

Nothing in this book should be considered medical advice. Always consult your doctor before making any changes to your diet, medical plan, exercise routine, or anything else that is important to your health. Be informed and make the best decision for *your* health!

Chapter #1
Change Your Habits To Change Your Life

"An ounce of prevention is worth a pound of cure."

Benjamin Franklin

"Good habits help you regain your health. Bad habits decrease the quality of your life. Choose your habits wisely."

Julie Luedtke

CHANGING YOUR HABITS IS ONE OF THE MOST difficult things you will do to increase the quality of your health.

If you think this is not important, just do a search on Google. There are over 200 *million* results for healthy habits.

And of course, the definition of habit is "a tendency or practice that is hard to give up."

I didn't have to look that up to figure it out.

How do we change the bad habits that are interfering with the quality of our life and replace them with good habits to increase our health?

It won't be easy, and some of your habits will be very difficult to change. But keep trying and never give up. Keep your focus on the goal of a healthy life. It will make the difference between quality of life after 55 or just plodding through each day.

Take some time to think about and write down your "WHY". Why is it important to you to be healthy?

Take a Simple Test

Here's a little test, similar to one we offered in the first book.

Sit in a comfortable chair without any distractions. Read Scene 1 and then close your eyes and imagine yourself in that position.

Scene 1. You are at the beach, sitting in the sand, watching your grandchild play along the edge of the water. A big wave knocks your grandchild off their feet and they scream for help.

You are unable to get to your feet quickly. You call out for someone to help the child, but no one can hear you. Your grandchild is crying and you are unable to get to your feet and help them.

How do you feel? Helpless? Fearful?

Now imagine yourself in a slightly different scenario.

Scene 2. You are at the beach, sitting in the sand, watching your grandchild play along the edge of the water. A big wave knocks your grandchild off their feet and they yell for help.

This time you scramble to your feet and rush to grab your precious grandchild, giving them a hug and comforting them. You are filled with gratitude that you were able to react quickly.

Now, you understand the importance of this book and the importance of changing bad habits into healthy ones.

This is the reason it is vital to take positive steps to live a healthy, vibrant life.

I could tell you that it would be easy to lose weight and be strong and healthy after 55. Just pop a few supplements and do a few exercises. Any weight loss or exercise plan will work if you stick to it. You will be healthy and active in 90 days.

Oh, I wish that was true!

How long does it take to break a bad habit?

Conventional wisdom says at least 21 days. That may be true for some people, but a habit will rear its ugly head in a matter of seconds under the right conditions.

Meet My Invisible Friends

Let me introduce you to the little gremlin sitting on my left shoulder and the charming angel on my right shoulder. The angel reminds me to stop eating sugar. I have tried for years to stop eating chocolate. Sometimes, I made it through the 21 days and thought, "Great! I've got that bad habit thrown out the window."

Then, I walk past the candy section of the grocery store, and the gremlin on my left shoulder gives a wicked chuckle. As if by magic, a package of chocolate candy jumps into my cart. And, yes, half the package is eaten before I even get home. The angel on my right shoulder just buries her head in her hands.

Am I the only one who has competing thoughts and temptations whispering in each ear? No!

What have I done to stop eating a half bag of chocolate candy during the 15 minute ride from the grocery store to my house?

Modify, Modify, Modify

I'm not saying it's the only method, but it will open up new ideas for you to change the bad habits in your life.

First, I limit the type of chocolate that I eat. I make sure it's dark chocolate and pieces are individually wrapped. I put the bag in a place that is not easily accessible, like the top shelf in the pantry … and make sure it is out of sight.

Then I set a goal. If I exercise five days in a row for at least 30 minutes, I can eat two pieces of chocolate. I make sure the calories in those two pieces of chocolate have been earned through working out. This is *not* a reward. It's just part of my goal.

Here's the amazing part. When I know that I can have the chocolate, and it's in the house, I don't crave it. When I have to work so hard to earn it, it loses its appeal.

It's Your Turn

Start to think about some of the habits you have that you know are not helping you regain or maintain your health.

Perhaps you just don't like to exercise. It's boring. You don't belong to a gym. You don't have clothes to wear.

Think about what you could do at home, wearing whatever clothes you already have.

Eliminate exercise from your thought process. Focus on *movement*. Do you like to putter in your garden? Set a goal of 30 minutes every other day. Do you watch television in the evening? Pull up a sturdy chair and practice the sit/stand movement later in this book during the commercials for one hour every other day. Is it too much movement? Modify until you accomplish your goal.

Think about what you will do every day to make healthy habits your priority and push the bad habits to the bottom of the list.

Those habits may not go away, but you minimize them and focus on the positive habits you are creating to live a healthier life.

When you start to waver, think back to the scenes at the beach. Which person do you want to be? Healthy and strong or weak and helpless?

Remember Your "WHY."

Just as in the first book *Healthy After 55, Live Your Best Life*, we will use acronyms to help you set your goals in each chapter.

H.A.B.I.T. is the logical acronym for this chapter. Get ready to push those unhealthy habits to the bottom of your list and create healthy new habits.

H is for Healthy
A is for Awareness
B is for Better
I is for Intentional
T is for Try, Try, Try Again

Step #1 — *Healthy*

Everything in this book is related to being healthy.

Habits are formed from choices you make.

Every time you reach for something to eat that isn't healthy, you are making a choice.

Every time you choose to move instead of sit in a chair, you are making a choice.

The more healthy choices you make, the more positive your habits become.

Step #2 — *Awareness is vital*

As you develop positive habits, be realistic.

Sometimes life is one big obstacle. Understand that you need to make the best choice for yourself at any given time. Be aware of what your choices really are at the moment.

You may not always make the best choice.

Before you reach for that candy bar or grab something at a fast food restaurant, ask yourself one question, "Will this make me healthier? Happier?"

The choice is yours.

Be aware of the choices you make and aim for more positive choices that will increase your health.

Step #3 — ***Better habits increase your health***

Those bad habits got you into this unhealthy lifestyle in the first place. Changing those habits one at a time will help you toward your goal of better health.

Think about a bad habit that you currently have. Maybe you sleep an extra 30 minutes rather than get up and exercise. Or perhaps you decide to have an unhealthy fast food dinner rather than make yourself a nutritious salad.

Pick one habit and make a conscious effort to change it *before you act on it*.

Put your workout clothes where you will see them when you wake up. Make the effort to get up and put those clothes on. Do whatever you had decided to do *before* going to sleep.

Before stopping at a fast food restaurant after work, have your healthy salad prepared at home and ready to eat. Or, better yet, choose a healthy food, if they have one, at the restaurant.

Take one step at a time.

Step #4 — ***Intentional choices will increase your healthy habits***

Making intentional choices is important if you want to regain and maintain your health.

All the charts in this book are designed to help you make intentional healthy choices.

When you print out the worksheet and complete the charts, you will be able to see your progress. You know what you need to do every day. You need to make intentional choices to complete the activities.

We've all heard the words, "If you fail to plan, you plan to fail." It is so true.

If I decide I want to complete a half marathon, I need to plan ahead. I need to know how many miles to walk/run each week, how long to go on a Saturday morning, and what to eat before, during and after long workouts. Then I put all the information on my calendar.

Disaster is assured if I think I can jump into my running shoes and complete 13.1 miles without a plan. Tried it once and it was ugly!

Make your movement and eating goals intentional. You will be making a giant leap in the right direction.

Step #5 — *Try, try, try again . . . never give up*

This is one of the most important components of changing bad habits into positive habits.

None of us are perfect. Life gets in the way of our best intentions. If we slip and fall once in a while, it does not mean we should stay down and forget about our healthy goals.

I've worked on improving my habits for more years than I can remember. There are times I find myself slipping back into unhealthy habits. After a few days, my energy evaporates and I realize how important movement and healthy eating are to my health and well-being.

Healthy habits are always a work in progress. Awareness and setting intentional goals are vital to that progress.

Use the worksheets at the end of each chapter to increase your success on this journey toward better healthy.

Print them out or go to our website HealthyAfter55.com to download and print the pdf copies at no charge.

Take time to complete them and save them. Refer back to worksheets you have completed when you feel yourself slipping into old habits.

Complete the first worksheet and post it where you will see it every day. Follow the steps for one week before moving on to the next chapter.

Introducing Your Accountability Buddy...

To add some zest to this adventure, meet your accountability buddy, Molly Wood.

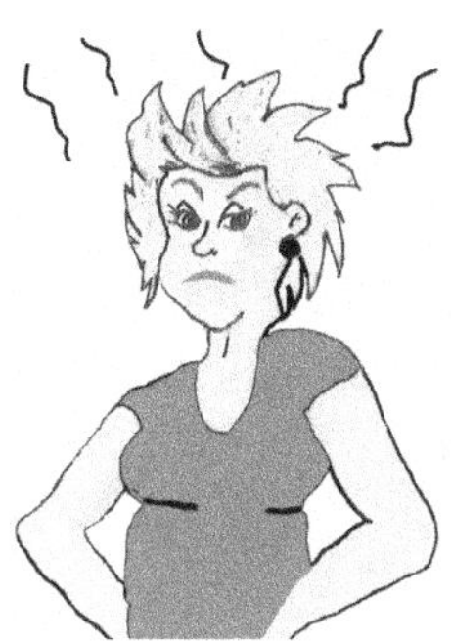

Molly will complete a sample of each worksheet and report her progress as she takes this journey with you.

Molly recently celebrated her 60th birthday. She is overweight, has high cholesterol, recently fell down and had difficulty getting back on her feet. She has one grandchild and loves to play with her, but has difficulty keeping up with the active 3-year-old. She secretly wonders if she will be able to play with her as she grows up.

Can you relate to Molly's concerns?

Worksheet for this chapter on Changing Habits

One habit you want to change _______________________________

Steps you will take to change that habit.

1. _______________________________
   ____

2. _______________________________
   ____

3. _______________________________
   ____

4. _______________________________
   ____

5. _______________________________
   ____

When you feel you have changed that habit, move on to another habit you want to change.

Continue to maintain the steps for the original habit as you build on your success.

This is an on-going process. Keep moving forward and … try, try, try again.

Molly's Plan to Change Her Habits

Molly had to think about her "WHY" for about five minutes. She wants to lose weight. Her first habit to break is eliminating her daily glass of wine … that often ended up being a bottle of wine after a particularly difficult day.

Steps to take to change her habit

1. Put the wine out of sight and have none in the fridge.

2. Take the wine glasses off the kitchen counter.

3. Take a walk after work to release the stress.

4. Try meditating for ten minutes after her walk.

5. Replace the wine after work with a cup of tea.

Stay tuned to see how this worked for her and meet her alter-ego, Hot Flash Holly.

What you learned in this chapter about Changing Habits.

You learned that it is important to change your habits for a healthy future. You need to do many things necessary for good health, but if you don't change your bad habits into positive ones, you set yourself up for failure.

- Start with one bad habit that is an obstacle in the path of your success to be healthy.

- Spend some time thinking of ways to change the negative habit into a positive routine.

- Remember your WHY.

- Almost is okay. No one is perfect.

- Keep trying to substitute healthy habits for the unhealthy habits you've spent a lifetime building up.

NOTE: If you have questions about anything in this book, do your research. Always consult your health care professional before making changes to your diet, medical plan, exercise routine, or anything else that is important to your health. Be informed. Take control. Make the best decision for your health!

Chapter #2
Right + Left = Balance

"Life is like riding a bicycle. To keep your balance, you must keep moving."

Albert Einstein

"Physical balance is important for quality of life. Done correctly, it will help strengthen your core and prevent falls."

Julie Luedtke

RIGHT NOW, YOU ARE PROBABLY SCRATCHING YOUR head and wondering, "What does balance have to do with eating healthy and movement?"

Balance Is Everything!

Balance is more than a fear of falling as you will discover in this book. It is more than exercise or movement. It is vital to your independence and quality of life.

When your balance is strong, you feel more like moving. You will be more confident walking and doing chores around the house. You will begin to see movement in a new light.

Think about it.

You need balance to do just about everything, every day. It includes: walking, getting out of a chair, and leaning over to tie your shoes, getting in and out of the shower, reaching for something on a top shelf, and stepping off the curb.

Strong muscles and the ability to keep yourself upright increase the quality of your life and contribute to your sense of well-being.

Stability Matters More Than Ever

When you were a child, you didn't want to fall because your peers would laugh at you. But if you fell down, you dusted yourself off, jumped up and kept going.

As you grow older, you become afraid of falling for more important reasons…broken bones, hospital stays, and loss of independence.

S.T.A.B.L.E. is an appropriate acronym for this chapter on balance. When you have stability in your stance and your walk, you feel better, stand up straighter, have more confidence in yourself, and have more energy.

Stability *is vital for your quality of life.*

S is for Start with one foot
T is for Test for 10 seconds
A is for Aim for 20 seconds
B is for Be aware
L is for Look straight ahead
E is for Evaluate

Step #1 — *Start with one foot*

Note: Before starting, make sure you check with your healthcare professional to insure that you don't have any health issues that might prevent you from doing this properly. If you have health issues that make you unsteady, ask them for guidance to make you stronger and increase your balance. This is for your health, not to hurt you.

Now … take one minute to check your balance.

To begin, wear comfortable shoes. Stand close to a counter in your kitchen or next to a sturdy chair.

- Stand on your right foot and count slowly to 5.

- When you have to put your left foot down to balance, stop and write that number down.

- Switch to stand on your left foot and count slowly to 5.

- When you have to put your right foot down to balance, stop and write that number down.

If you were able to count to 5 without touching the counter or chair while balancing on either foot, congratulations!

Try it with bare feet. If you were still able to count to 5 while standing on each foot, move on to the next step.

Having Trouble Balancing?

- Keep your head up and stand as straight as possible.

- Focus on an object about 10 feet in front of you at eye level.

- Slowly lift your arms out to your sides before lifting your leg.

- Raise one foot just a few inches off the ground so you can put it down quickly.

- Continue to practice several times a day until you are able balance on each foot. Remember to wear comfortable shoes before trying it with bare feet.

Then move on to the next step.

Step #2 — *Test for 10 seconds*

When you were able to count to 5, you are ready for this step.

Wear comfortable shoes before starting. Stand close to a counter in your kitchen or a sturdy chair.

- Stand on your right foot and count slowly to 10. Write that number down.

- Switch and stand on your left foot and count slowly to 10. Write that number down.

- If you were able to count to 10 without touching the counter or chair when balancing on either foot, congratulations!

Try it with bare feet before moving on to the next step.

Having Trouble Balancing?

If you counted to less than 10, you need to work on your strength and balance to prevent falling.

- Keep your head up and stand as straight as possible.

- Focus on an object about 10 feet in front of you at eye level.

- Slowly lift your arms out to your sides before lifting your leg.

- Bend your knee and raise one foot just a few inches off the ground so you can put it down quickly if necessary.

Continue to work on this step until you are able to balance on each leg for 10 seconds in shoes and in bare feet before moving on to Step 3.

Step #3 — *Aim for 20 seconds*

If you were able to count to 10, you are ready to try this step.

Again, wear comfortable shoes before starting.

- Stand close to a counter in your kitchen or a sturdy chair.

- Stand on your right foot and see if you can count slowly to 20. Write that number down.

- Stand on your left foot and count slowly to 20. Write that number down.

If you were able to count to 20 without touching the counter or chair when balancing on either foot, congratulations!

Try it with bare feet before moving on to the next step.

Continue to work on this step until you can balance on each leg for 20 seconds in shoes and in bare feet before moving on to Step 4.

Note: You were probably able to balance on one foot longer than the other. That's because we all have a dominant side that is stronger than the less dominant side. It's important to increase the strength on your non-dominant side to keep you upright and …balanced.

After that little experiment, you might start to think about your balance and a strong core with more interest.

What Is Core Strength? Why Is It Important?

We talk about core strength throughout this book because it *is* important. Your core keeps you upright and promotes a healthy back, helps you stand up without help after sitting, and keeps the blood moving through your body.

Note: Do a search on the internet and you will find hundreds of websites that guarantee a stronger core in 30 days. Be very careful. Many of the exercises shown are difficult and put a strain on your back and neck. The person demonstrating the exercise is usually under the age of 40 with zero percent body fat. Core strength is important for your health, not to cause injury.

Your core strength starts with your abdominal muscles. When you stand up straight and try to touch your navel to your spine, you are using your core muscles.

When you try to stand up using your hips and thighs instead of your hands, you are using your core muscles.

When you start to fall down and are able to catch yourself and return to a stand, you are using your core muscles.

You will understand why your core is so important.

We will show you core exercises that are meant to help you. They can be done in the comfort of your home without any expensive equipment.

Balance and Your Brain

Balance coordinates the use of your muscles with your brain. You need both your brain and your body to work together to react quickly if you start to fall.

Practicing balance is necessary to maintain not only the quality of your health, but your confidence as well.

True Story

A 77-year-old gentleman in my exercise class told me that the previous day he stumbled at home and started to fall forward. He had fallen several months earlier and injured his wrist, so he started to panic.

Without thinking about it, his left leg quickly moved forward and then his right leg and he regained his balance. He said the balance exercises we did in class saved him from falling down.

What a difference a simple exercise made not only to his confidence, but also to the quality of his life!

Step #4 — *Be aware*

Be aware that a strong core will help to keep you balanced and upright.

When you are standing in line at the grocery store, stand up straight and try to connect your belly button with your spine. Count to 10 and release. Continue to do this simple exercise as long as you are in line.

Here are some additional movements that will help improve your stability and may help to prevent falls. They strengthen your legs and core while helping your brain remember what to do if you start to lose your balance.

Try This At Home

While you are waiting for something to heat up in the microwave

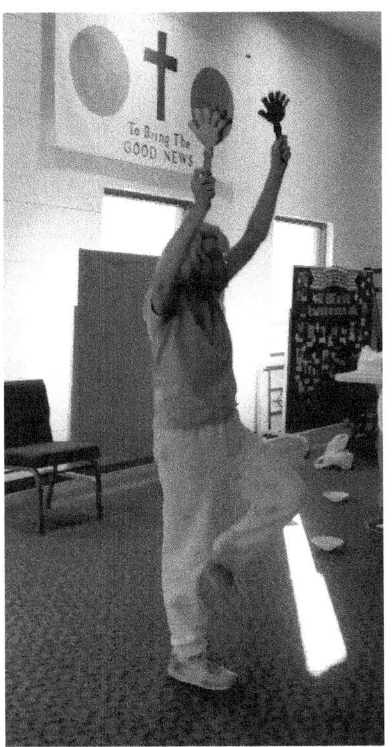

In my classes I find fun ways to practice balance.

- Stand close to a counter or wall, stand on one foot and focus at least 10 feet in front of you for 30 seconds.

- Then stand on the other foot for 30 seconds. You will find it is easier to balance with shoes on, and one foot will be easier to balance on than the other.

- Once you do this movement easily, try it with your eyes closed! Make sure you stand close to a counter or wall to catch yourself if you start to wobble.

Step #5 — ***Look straight ahead***

Single Leg Lift

- Single Leg Life is a movement to strengthen your legs and core.

- Stand next to a sturdy chair or wall, with your right hand on the chair or wall.

- Look straight ahead.

- Use your core to keep your body upright and slowly lift your left leg straight out in front of you as far as you are able while maintaining your balance.

- Bring that leg back down.

- Lift your leg to the side only as far as you are able while maintaining your balance

- Bring your leg back down.

- Lift the same leg slightly to the back.

- Return to your original position.

Do this exercise 10 times and switch to the other leg.

When you can do it easily, try it without holding onto the chair.

Try the Sobriety Test

This series of movements is a favorite in my exercise classes. They named this exercise the "Sobriety Test".

- Put your right heel in front of your left toe; continue with your left heel in front of your right foot … as if you were walking on a tightrope.

- Have your arms out to your sides at shoulder level.

- Focus on a spot approximately 10 feet in front of you.

- Stay close to a counter or wall if you need to catch yourself. Go forward 15–20 steps

- Turn around and go back to where you started.

When you are able to do this exercise without your arms out for balance, try it with your arms at your sides. When you get really good at it, try it backward.

This is a student in class using her arms for balance and doing the Sobriety Test.

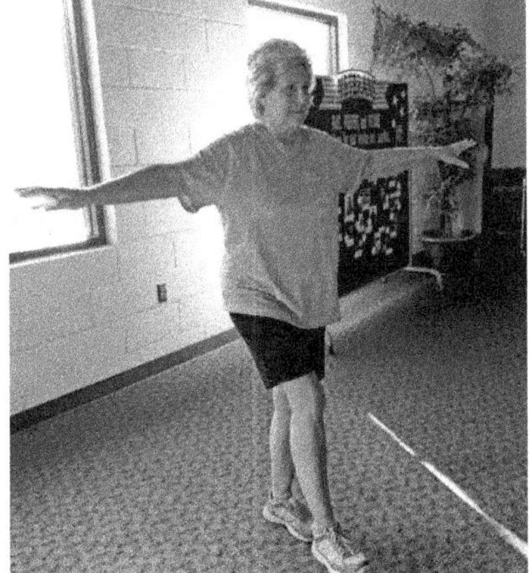

Try Communication – Your Legs and Brain

Help your brain remember what to tell your body to do if you start to fall.

- Stand next to a sturdy chair with your right hand on it.

- Lift your left leg slightly.

- Push it forward as if you were going to take a big step and step down.

Do this 10 times with your left leg.

- Stand next to a sturdy chair with your left hand on it.

- Lift your right leg slightly.

- Push it forward as if you were going to take a big step and step down.

When you can take a step forward easily with either leg, do it to the side with each leg.

Step # 6 — *Evaluate*

It's time to evaluate what you have learned in this chapter on balance.

Here is a worksheet to help you evaluate where you are and what you want to accomplish.

You will find these movements and others to help your balance on our Facebook page: Facebook.com/Healthy After55

PDF copies of the worksheets are located on our website: HealthyAfter55.com Feel free to print and use them as needed.

Worksheet for this chapter on Balance

Check off each movement when you are able to do it correctly every day for one week. Continue to do these simple moves until they become a positive habit.

Single Leg Life

☐ Stand next to counter. Balance on right foot for 30 seconds. When you can do it with your eyes open, close your eyes and do it.

☐ Stand next to counter. Balance on left foot for 30 seconds. When you can do it with your eyes open, close your eyes and do it.

☐ Stand with right hand on sturdy chair or counter. Life left leg slowly to the front, then the side, and then the back. Switch sides

Sobriety Test

☐ Walk toe-to-heel in a straight line for 25 steps. Turn around and to back to start.

☐ Walk toe-to-heel in a straight line for 25 steps backward.

Communication – Your Legs and Brain

☐ Stand with right hand on sturdy chair or counter. Lift left leg out in front of you, and then step down. Repeat 10 times.

☐ Stand with right hand on sturdy chair or counter. Lift left leg out to the side of you, and then step down. Repeat 10 times.

☐ Stand with left hand on sturdy chair or counter. Lift right leg out in front of you, and then step down. Repeat 10 times.

☐ Stand with left hand on sturdy chair or counter. Lift right leg out to the side of you, and then step down. Repeat 10 times.

Molly Works on Her Balance

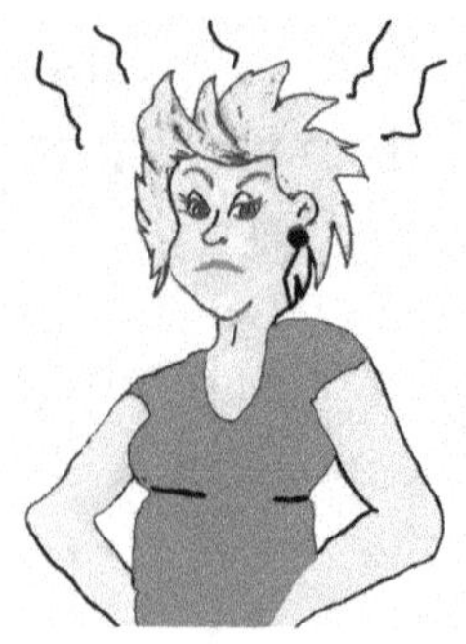

This wasn't as easy as she thought it would be.

SINGLE LEG LIFT

Molly was able to balance on her right foot for 20 seconds, but didn't last 15 seconds on her left foot.

She forgot that one side of her body was stronger than the other. She had to work on her left side.

It took a week of doing it every day before she could do it for 30 seconds.

It took another week before she even tried it with her eyes closed.

SOBRIETY TEST

This was even more difficult for Molly. She began to wonder if she could ever walk a straight line even when she was sober.

Now it's time to meet her alter-ego, Hot Flash Holly.

Hot Flash Holly entered Molly's life when the hot flashes kept Molly awake at night and when she wondered if she should even bother trying to regain her health. Was it worth the effort?

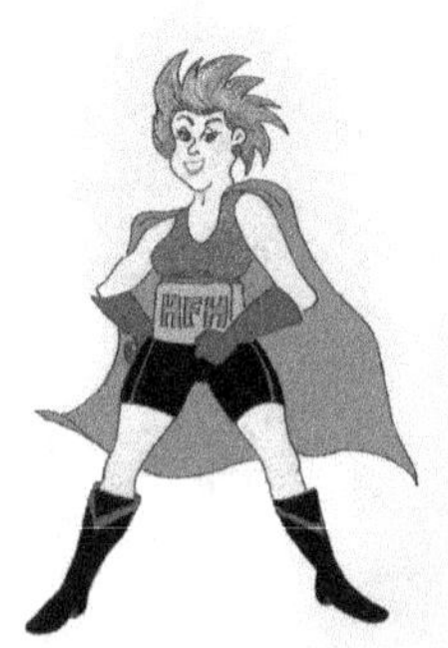

Hot Flash Holly sat on Molly's shoulder and encouraged her to take small steps and work toward better health.

Molly started with ten steps, increased it to 15 steps, then 20 steps and finally 25 steps. It took her a couple of weeks of practicing every day, but she gave herself a pat on the back when she accomplished her goal … even though she thought about a glass of wine to celebrate. She realized the irony of that thought and gave a nod to Hot Flash Holly.

COMMUNICATION – LEGS AND BRAIN

That seemed like a weird title for an exercise on balance, but Molly thought she might as well give it a try.

How hard could it be?

The kitchen counter caught her several times before she lost her balance.

This exercise took her a little longer to accomplish her goal, but within three weeks, she was able to do it without reaching for the kitchen counter.

Hot Flash Holly approved.

What you learned in this chapter about Balance.

You learned that balance is important for your overall health. Balance is something you don't think about, but it is vital to your quality of life.

- Doing simple movements every day will increase your balance, and also strengthen your core.

- As your balance becomes better, your fear of falling will decrease.

- Balance movements can be done anytime, anywhere.

- Balance is an excellent way to begin to regain your health and increase the quality of your life.

NOTE: If you have questions about anything in this book, do your research. Always consult your health care professional before making changes to your diet, medical plan, exercise routine, or anything else that is important to your health. Be informed. Take control. Make the best decision for your health!

Chapter #3
Stir The Pot

"Movement should be approached like life-enthusiasm, joy and gratitude—for movement is life, and life is movement, and we get out of it what we put into it."

Ron Fletcher

*"By moving for just 20 minutes a day, you may decrease your chance for a stroke or heart attack . . . **and** When you add some moderate strength training you may increase your life expectancy. Most importantly, you will increase the quality of your life!"*

Julie Luedtke

EVERYONE KNOWS THAT MOVEMENT IS GOOD FOR your health. But did you know it's also good for your mood **and** your brain?

Getting Started – How Hard Will It Be?

If you are reading this book, you know one of the biggest problems with any kind of movement or exercise is getting started. Maybe you have some apps on your smart phone or tablet that show all these great exercises … except most of them are led by someone in their 20's with zero percent body fat. They do the exercises easily and quickly, leaving you frustrated, confused and irritated.

I've been there. I understand.

All of the movements and exercises in this book can be done in your own home and at your own speed. The examples you see are either me or one of my classes demonstrating the moves.

See For Yourself
Check the demonstration videos on my Facebook page, Healthy After 55.

If 20 minutes sounds like a long time, break it into 5 or 10 minute segments and then gradually add more time. It all begins with one step.

Stop Making Excuses!
There isn't an excuse I haven't heard.

- "It's too hot (or cold) to go outside. There isn't anything I can do in the house."

- "I don't like to exercise."

- "I don't want to pay for an expensive gym."

- "I don't have clothes to wear."

- "I can't find my shoes."

- "I don't have any equipment."

- "I'm too old, too overweight, or too sore."

No more excuses! There are simple movements in this book that anyone is able to do at home.

NOTE: *If anything hurts, don't do it! Always check with your health care professional before starting any exercise program.*

Are you ready to improve your strength and health?

Jessica's story...

I told this story in the first book, but it's important to repeat it.

I led the corporate wellness challenge at a company where I worked. Jessica, an overweight woman in her early 50's shyly approached me and said that she would like to start walking to lose some weight, but even a mile was too much for her.

I showed her how to use a simple pedometer. We started with a reasonable number of steps she was able to do in a day and then a week. She slowly increased the steps she took every day, and within two months, she had lost 12 pounds and was feeling more confident and ready to move to the next level in her personal wellness.

By the time we did another wellness challenge a year later, she had lost 105 pounds, had more confidence, and was happier and healthier!

Her journey to achieve health and happiness was accomplished ... *one step at a time.*

This may not be easy. It's possible you've tried other programs and after a few weeks or maybe even a couple of months, you started to miss a few days, then a week, and then forgotten it completely.

This book is about changing your habits and lifestyle so these simple tips will become part of your daily routine.

If you read the first book in the series *Healthy After 55 – Live Your Best Life*, you will see that the goals we set in the first book carry over into this book.

Are you beginning to see the pattern for a healthy lifestyle?

Remember your "WHY".

B.E.G.I.N. is the logical acronym for this chapter. Get ready to move forward, one step at a time.

B is for Better every day
E is for Excuses be gone
G is for Get started
I is for It's never too late
N is for Now is the time

Step #1 – *Better every day*

Just take one step and build slowly. Every day will get better when you make the effort to *move*.

Here is an easy way to get started in your own home.

Stand Up, Sit Down, One More Time

- Sit on a solid chair (kitchen or dining room chair)

- Focus on using your thighs and your core to sit and stand

- Without using your hands, stand up

- Sit down, count to 5

- Stand up again

Practice this until you are able to do it during an entire commercial on television.

When you are able to complete this exercise through one commercial, try doing it through a second commercial, until you are able to do it through all the commercials in a half hour show.

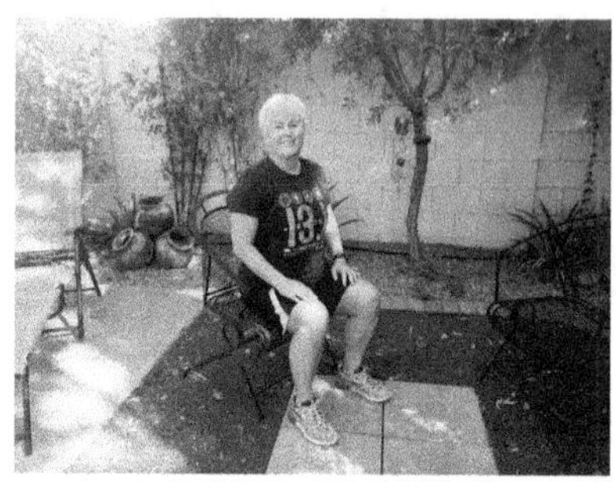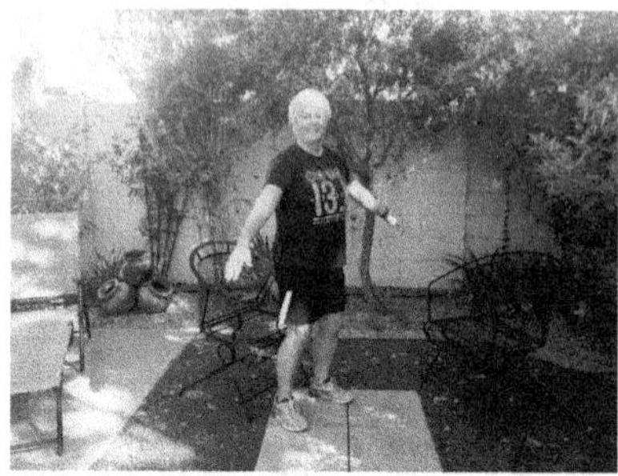

Sit on a sturdy chair then stand without using your hands.
I like to practice this movement in my backyard.

Step #2 – *Excuses be gone*

Understand your goals, identify potential obstacles, and *modify* them as necessary.

Banish all the excuses that prevent you from moving.

Remember the scenario in the introduction? Do you want to be healthy and strong or weak and helpless? Remember your "WHY".

Set goals that work for you. If your goal is to walk a mile, start with a walk around the block. If your goal is to have better balance, do the movement patterns in Chapter 2.

Keep moving forward and ignore those excuses.

Joanne's Story

One of the ladies I worked with, Joanne, had a difficult time doing any of the things I suggested on the days when we didn't meet.

At one of our sessions I had her tell me about some of the things she loved to do and what motivated her to do them. She loved to quilt and showed me photos of beautiful designs she created.

I suggested she use her calendar, set a goal each day to complete one set of movements, and when she accomplished that goal, she could begin quilting.

Joanne not only started setting and accomplishing her movement goals, but she made several beautiful placemats, and gave two of them to me when she lost ten pounds. What a great win-win for both of us.

Step #3 – *Get started*

This may be the most challenging part of any lifestyle change.

When you fall off the wagon it is important to stand up straight, dust yourself off and resume your movement schedule. The effort will be worth the quality of life that you are creating for yourself. No one will do it for you. This is something that only you can do.

- Take a deep breath, close your eyes, and remember "WHY" you started reading this book. You first pictured in your mind's eye the inability to get off the sand to save your grandchild who was overcome by a wave. Then you pictured yourself being capable of getting up and reaching them before any harm could be done. That took effort and you need to keep that feeling to maintain the effort.

- Buy some fun stickers and put one on your calendar every day you do some physical movement. It could be gardening, cleaning the house, taking a walk in the neighborhood, parking your car a little farther away from the store, playing with your children, taking a pet for a walk, or dancing around the house. Any physical movement. When you make it something you like to do, you will be more likely to continue doing it.

Step #4 – *It's never too late*

Remind yourself of the reasons you want to do this. You are doing this not only yourself, but also for your loved ones.

Pull out the list of reasons why it's important for you to increase the quality of your life.

Add more reasons to that list as you think of why your health is a priority.

Do you have friends who need to regain their health? Start a support group. Meet one day a week to walk and set goals. Have fun. Laugh and enjoy the comradery.

Step #5 – *Now is the time*

Ask yourself, "If not now, when?"

When will you take the first step toward a healthy lifestyle? Tomorrow? Next week? Next month?

Be realistic. You are an older adult. You may have difficulty climbing a flight of stairs or lifting a bag of groceries.

How long are you going to wait to begin your journey toward a healthier, happier life?

If not now, when?

No more excuses!

Here are some simple movements to do at home.

NOTE: *Please! If anything hurts, don't do it! Always check with your health care professional before starting any exercise program or trying anything new. This is for your health.*

- Turn on some music. Find something that you like, that makes you think about something fun when you were young. Start moving to the music (if your neighbors see you, so much the better!)

- Don't want to dance? Pretend you are the conductor and wave your arms.

- Do you have a garden or plants that need watering and trimming? Bending over to pull out weeds is a great way to move. Just make sure to "hinge" from your hips, keep your back flat and your head in line with your back. It will take the pressure off your lower back. Please visit my Facebook page (Healthy After 55) for a video on an easy way to pick something up off the floor or ground.

- Walk around a room or your yard while alternating knee lifts with each step, raising the opposite arm at the same time. When you can do it easily, try doing it raising your arm and leg on the same side.

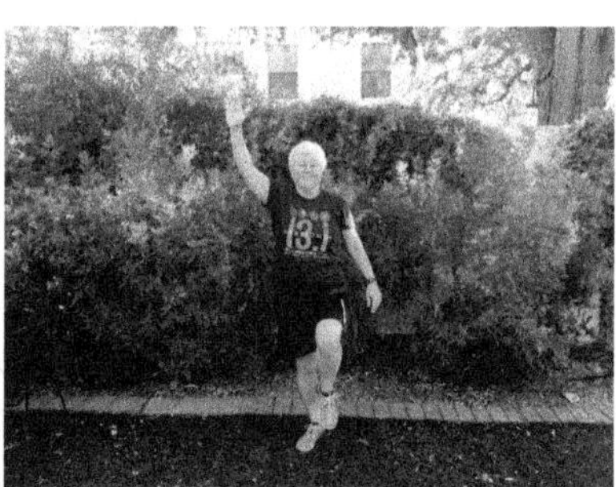

Alternating knee lifts while raising the opposite arm. Doing this in my backyard amuses my neighbors.

- Sit on a chair with both feet on the floor, slowly raise one foot about 6 inches off the floor and hold it to the count of 10. Slowly put it back on the floor. Repeat 10 times. Switch to the other leg.

- Park next to the shopping cart drop off when you go grocery shopping. Walk down every aisle at the store before checking out. You will be surprised at how many minutes you are active.

More about Jessica

A year after that first wellness challenge Jessica had lost over 100 pounds. She not only had more confidence, but she was happier and healthier! Jessica went back to school and got her degree. She was ready to move on. She landed a job she had dreamed about for a long time and moved across the country to start a new life.

We stayed in touch and Jessica has continued to set more goals for herself. She completed her first marathon just a few months ago and sent me a photo of herself, a big smile on her face as she held up her medal after finishing the race.

Jessica achieved health and happiness ...*one step at a time.*

Resistance training is a good way to strengthen your muscles.

You know resistance training is a good way to strengthen your muscles, but you may not want to go to a gym or are afraid of injuring yourself.

Here are easy exercises done with a bath towel while you watch TV. You can see demonstrations of these exercises and others on our Facebook page.

Scratch Your Back

Use a bath towel or beach towel.

- Grasp one end of your bath towel with your left hand and wrap the towel around your back.

- Grasp the other end of the towel with your right hand.

- Pull on the towel with both hands while standing tall.

- Hold it for a count of 10.

- Relax and do it again.

- Repeat it 5 times.

- Gradually increase the amount of time you are able to keep resistance on the towel.

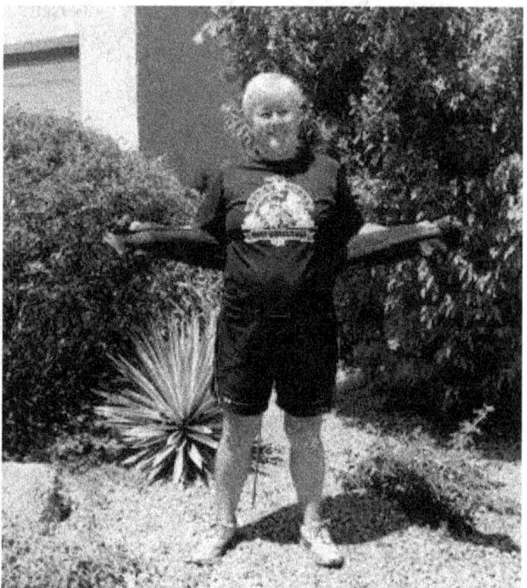

Scratch Your Back – Pull on the towel while you stand tall.

- This strengthens your core, back, grip, fingers and wrists.

Pull the Towel Apart

- Grasp the ends of the towel with your hands and try to pull the towel apart.

- Raise your right hand and pull

- Raise your left hand and pull.

- This is a great exercise to strengthen your grip, wrists and arms without putting too much pressure on your joints.

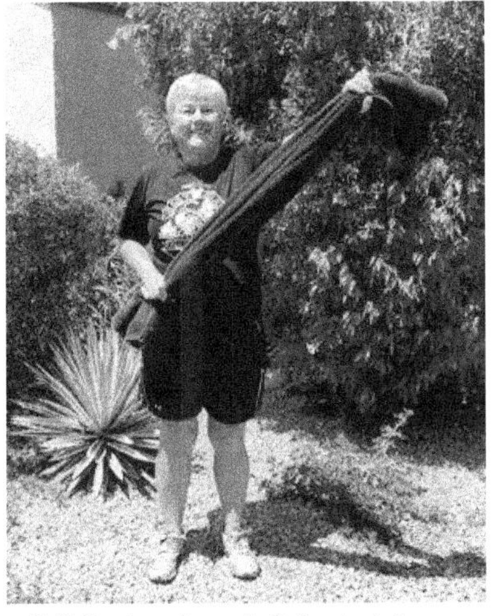

Pull the towel apart. Only stretch your arms out to a comfortable distance.

Toe Stretch

- Sit down on a chair

- Grasp the towel in both hands and slide it under your right foot.

- Keep your back and leg straight.

- Pull on the towel.

- Repeat with your left leg.

- When this is easy to do, raise your leg slightly when you pull on the towel.

No weights for strength training? No problem.

There are easy ways to increase your strength without going to the gym or buying expensive equipment.

Do this movement when you are at the park watching your children or grandchildren play a sport. Use a couple of water bottles (good way to remember to drink water). When they are empty, fill them with small stones or sand to add a little weight. (Unopened soup cans also work when you do these exercises at home.)

Arm Curls

- Hold one bottle in each hand, palms up.

- Slowly curl one arm up, keeping your elbow at your side.

- Hold it for a count of 5 and then slowly return your hand to your side.

- Repeat 5 times with one arm.

- Switch to the other arm.

- When you can do it easily, do both arms at the same time, and increase the count to 10, 15, 20.

Banish the Bat Wings

- Hold one bottle in your right hand, your arm at your side.

- Push your hand back until you feel the tension in the back of your upper arm. Hold it for a count of 5.

- Slowly return your arm to your side.

- Repeat 5 times

- Do the same movement with your left arm.

- When you can do it easily, do both arms at the same time and increase the count to 10, 15, 20.

Take Time to Chill Out

- When you feel stressed, take several deep breaths.

- Take a deep breath in through your nose

- Count to 5

- Exhale through your mouth.

- Do this 3–5 times and relax.

*Move more for a happier, healthier **you.***

Bonus movement

I'm on the floor . . . how do I get back on my feet?

This is the best way to get up off the floor if you have difficulty standing without help.

- Roll to your hands and knees

- Place your dominant foot on the floor in front of you with your knee up.

- Put your hand on that thigh

- Curl the toes of your back foot

- Push up with the toes of your back foot.

A video of this exercise is on our Facebook page: Facebook.com /HealthyAfter55

One of my students was excited to learn about this technique to stand up. She laughed and said it was the first time she could get up off the floor without help after playing with her grandchildren. Her family was impressed.

Worksheet for this chapter on How To Start Moving

NOTE: Before starting this or any exercise program, make sure to discuss your options with your health care professional. Take this book with you or show them the Facebook page and follow their guidance on what you should do and what you should avoid or modify.

When you start this program, do these movements once a week for the first couple of weeks. If you feel ok, increase to twice a week, then three times a week.

If you feel any pain or soreness, stop doing that movement and wait a couple of days before starting again.

The key is to continue to *move* to build your strength and then maintain it. This is for your health, not to hurt you.

Each day write down what movement you did and the effort you put into it on a scale of 1–5

Scratch Your Back

Arm curls

Pull the Towel Apart

Banish the Bat Wings

Toe Stretch

Take Time to Chill

Scale for effort

    1 = no effort, just rolled out of bed

    2 = not breathing hard

    3 = starting to breath hard, a little sweaty

    4 = working up a sweat, breathing hard

    5 = difficult to finish, but you did it!

	Effort	Effort	Effort	Effort	Effort	Effort	Effort
Scratch Your Back							
Pull Towel Apart							
Toe Stretch							
Arm Curl							
Banish Bat Wings							
Take Time to Chill Out							

For videos of these movements and additional easy movements you are able to do at home, please visit my Facebook page HealthyAfter55.

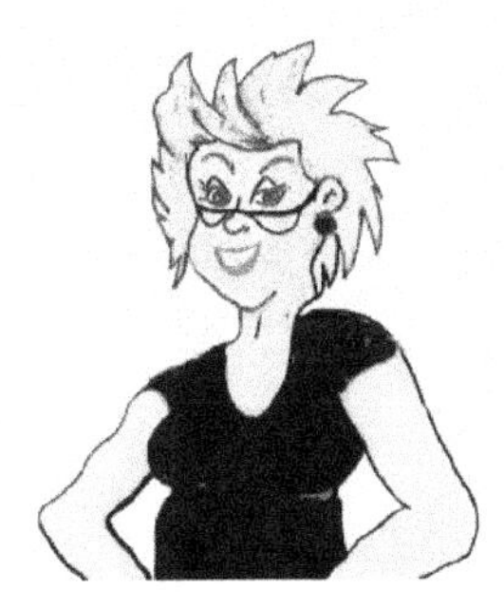

Molly Wood thought this would be easy … until she came home from a stressful day at work and was exhausted.

Hot Flash Holly sat on her shoulder as she looked longingly at the bottle of wine in her wine rack.

"Molly, Molly, Molly." Hot Flash murmured. "You took a big step toward regaining your health. Do you want to give up now?"

Taking a deep breath, Molly started with Take Time to Chill Out.

That wasn't too bad, so she put on her pajamas, grabbed a bath towel and did Scratch Your Back. Her effort was a 3, but she did it and moved on to the next movement.

She thought of several people at work as she did Pull the Towel Apart. That earned her an effort of 5.

The Toe Stretch was an effort of 3, but the Arm Curls were an effort of 4 and she really wanted to Banish the Bat Wings, so that earned her an effort of 5.

Molly didn't try the bonus of getting up off the floor. She thought she might end up sleeping on the floor rather than trying to stand up.

Hot Flash Holly gave her a thumbs up for her effort before Molly collapsed into bed.

What you learned in this chapter on How to Start Moving.

You learned that it is important to take that first step toward physical movement. You do all the other things necessary for good health, but if you neglect movement, you set yourself up for failure.

- Start with one step and keep moving forward

- Take your time as you make this important lifestyle change

- Effort is important to maintain your new movement goals

- Purpose will keep you focused as you remember the reason WHY you want to be healthy

NOTE: If you have questions about anything in this book, do your research. Always consult your health care professional before making changes to your diet, medical plan, exercise routine, or anything else that is important to your health. Be informed. Take control. Make the best decision for your health!

Chapter #4
Step It Up

"Movement is the song of the body."

Vanda Scaravelli

"It's time to make your body sing and move!"

Julie Luedtke

IT'S TIME TO MAKE SOME IMPORTANT DECISIONS.

Think about the goals you want to accomplish. We've talked about eliminating bad habits and starting healthy habits.

Now is the time to begin to regain your health. Begin your journey... one step at a time.

Getting Ready

Before you begin, identify potential obstacles. Talk to your health care professional and make sure that a walking program is good for your health. Discuss any injuries or movement issues... back, hips, knees, ankles, feet. If you have any problems, talk about alternative movements that will help you regain your health. Your health care professional is your partner in this journey. Utilize their expertise.

Once you are encouraged to start a walking plan, the first thing you need to do is make sure you have good, sturdy walking shoes. Trying to walk any distance in sandals or old worn out sneakers is a sure way to create sore muscles and injuries. This will decrease your chances for success.

Wear comfortable clothing that is weather-appropriate if you are going to walk outside. If the weather is too hot or cold, go to a mall and walk for 30 minutes. Take the stairs if possible.

Purchase an inexpensive pedometer (available in the Sporting Goods Department at most stores) or use your smartphone with an app to track how many steps you take during the day (this works if you keep your phone in your pocket all day). Do some research to see which app is best for you.

I personally use a Fitbit™. It's a little more expensive than just a pedometer. Fitness trackers measure everything from steps, to goal setting, calories burned, and fitness activity. The added motivation for me is if it costs more money than a pedometer, I will use it every day to get my money's worth.

Once you have a way to track your steps, see how many steps you average every day for a week. Write the number down every day and add them up.

This is the time to be honest with yourself. See how many steps you take during a day. Numbers don't lie.

When it comes to movement, **S.T.E.P.** is the logical acronym for this chapter and a great way to remember to move.

S is for Start
T is for Take your time
E is for Effort
P is for Purpose

Step #1 – *Start*

This is the hardest part. Take that first step and build slowly. Use your pedometer or Fitbit or an app to help you get started. It's not important where you start …it's more important to move and improve.

Remember that everyone who has been successful at regaining and maintaining their health had to start where you are …with that first step.

Put your start date on your calendar in big, bold letters. Be proud that you decided to take control of your health.

Remember your "WHY" when you decided it was time to regain your health.

That's your motivation to start moving. One step at a time …

Step # 2 – *Take your time*

It took you some years to get out of shape, so be realistic. It will take time to regain your health. Just as it takes time to build a strong building, it takes time to build a strong body.

If you try to do too much, too soon, you will set yourself up for failure. Your goal is a healthy lifestyle for the rest of your life. And that, my friend, takes time.

This is a lifestyle change and you will set goals, get off track, and need to adjust your goals and restart. A healthy lifestyle is your journey. *You control what you do and when you do it.*

The important thing to remember – *don't give up!*

Step #3 – *Effort*

I can't stress this enough. Without effort on your part, this won't happen. I can't do this for you. I will encourage you and give you the steps that need to be taken to regain your health. However, the only person who is able to regain your health is *you!*

You probably thought that reading this book was enough effort to make you healthy again …and live happily ever after. Both are fairy tales that never happen in real life.

It takes *effort* to get out of bed in the morning and take a walk before work.

It takes *effort* to take a walk after work when you'd rather sit in front of the television.

It takes *effort* to walk on a Saturday morning instead of sleeping an extra 30 minutes.

You know where this is going …*it takes effort to accomplish anything worthwhile, and creating a healthy lifestyle for yourself is definitely worthwhile.*

Step #4 – ***Purpose***

Remember "WHY" you started this journey to improve your health.

Look at what you've already accomplished in your life and what you want to accomplish in the future.

Look at your children or grandchildren. How important is it to you to be able to go on family vacations, play with them, and enjoy doing things with them?

Think about how amazed they will be when you go to the pumpkin farm and bend over, pick up a pumpkin and hand it to them!

Worksheet for this chapter as you take your first STEPS toward a healthy lifestyle

Week 1. Record how many steps you take each day.

Week 2. Increase the steps you recorded from Week 1. It doesn't make any difference how many steps you increase, just increase them and write them down.

Week 3. Increase the steps you recorded in Week 2 by 25 steps every day.

Week 4. Increase your steps from Week 3 by 50 steps every day.

	M	T	W	T	F	S	S
Week 1							
Week 2							
Week 3							
Week 4							

During the next four weeks, increase your steps every day. It doesn't matter how many you do or how you do them, just increase them every day. If you need a break, take one day of rest every week. You earned it!

	M	T	W	T	F	S	S
Week 5							
Week 6							
Week 7							
Week 8							

Molly decided to invest in a FitBit™ to help her track her steps. She thought this would be an easy step. After all, she was always walking around at work.

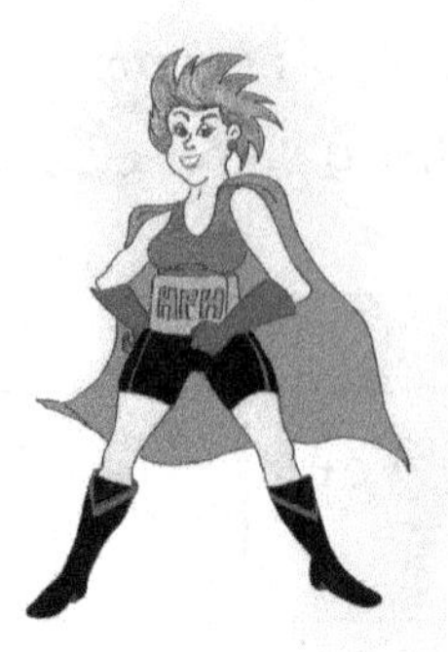

She faithfully recorded her steps during Week 1 and was surprised that she didn't walk as much as she thought she did.

Week 2 she walked a few more steps each day, but it was an effort. She made a few more trips to the restroom at work and took the steps instead of the elevator to the second floor, but there wasn't a big change in her step count.

Week 3 she had to walk around the yard to add extra steps to each day and by Week 4, she knew she would have to make a few more changes.

Molly bought some new walking shoes and started to wear them after work. She started to walk around the block and met neighbors she hadn't seen before.

Week 5 was hectic at work and her step count decreased. By Saturday, she covered her head with her pillow and decided to sleep instead of going for a walk.

Hot Flash Holly started to hop on the pillow and hopped all over Molly. "Get up! You need to move! You've come too far to stop now. You just bought new shoes. Use them!"

Molly knew she wouldn't get any more sleep, so she stumbled out of bed, got dressed and went for a walk. She was surprised she had walked so far and felt much better than when she started.

Maybe counting steps and walking would be better than she expected it to be.

What you learned in this chapter about taking the first Steps toward a healthy lifestyle.

You learned that it is important to take that first step toward movement. You do all the other things necessary for good health, but if you neglect movement, you set yourself up for failure.

- Start with one step and keep moving forward

- Take your time as you make this important lifestyle change

- Effort is important to maintain your movement toward your goals

- Purpose will keep you focused as you remember "why" your health is important

NOTE: If you have questions about anything in this book, do your research. Always consult your health care professional before making changes to your diet, medical plan, exercise routine, or anything else that is important to your health. Be informed. Take control. Make the best decision for your health!

Chapter #5
Food Fight!

Diet is a Four-Letter Word
Eliminate the word "diet" and focus on "Eating Well"

"If you want to change your body, you need to change how you think about food. Food is fuel for your body, not therapy."

Julie Luedtke

YOU PROBABLY *KNEW* THAT, BUT *DOING* SOMETHING about it is more difficult to accomplish. Changing your relationship with food is one of the most challenging steps you will take.

If you looked through the book, saw the chapter on diet, and decided to jump ahead to this chapter, you will be disappointed.

If you expected a miracle announcement to help you lose weight while eating whatever you want to …it's not going to happen.

Diet really is a four letter word. You are bombarded with ads regarding what to eat and how to lose weight every day. Some make sense. Others are difficult to follow for more than a day or two and are forgotten in a week.

Most diets are not lifestyle changers

If you are like me, you've tried more weight loss programs than you even remember. One of my more memorable weight loss experiments was a seminar involving hypnosis and imagining your favorite food covered in worms … that did not work so well. Instead of turning off the desire for food, my friend and I giggled way too much and stopped for pizza and a glass of wine when the seminar ended.

Many of us have lived the "food fight" all of our lives! You start another diet with high hopes; lose a couple of pounds, and then life gets in the way … AGAIN! You gain the weight back plus a few more pounds and inches. *And* it gets more difficult with each passing year.

After menopause, it gets worse. You pull up your granny pants, plop down in front of the television and feel sorry for yourself with a bowl of ice cream.

Have you ever said …

"Why should I bother changing my eating habits now?"

"I'm too old to change what I eat."

"It's just part of nature to gain weight after menopause. Why should I fight it?"

"No matter what I do, it won't make any difference."

Just like every other positive step you take for a healthier, happier life, this will be a challenge and it will take effort.

It is never too late to start eating for a healthy life

This chapter is going to give you some tips to start moving forward on your journey toward a healthy lifestyle.

It makes sense that the acronym for healthy eating would be **F.O.O.D.**

F is for *Follow a healthy eating plan*
O is for *Ounces of water*
O is for *Out of sight, out of mind*
D is for *Don't dwell on mistakes*

Step #1: *Follow a healthy eating plan*

- Eating well is an important part of your plan to regain and maintain your health. Find a qualified nutritionist who understands your health issues. They help you create an eating plan that will work for years to come, not just a few weeks.

- Find an app for your smart phone to help you track what you eat every day. There are plenty of apps available. Find one that is motivating and will keep you focused on your goal. My personal favorites are *Lose It!*™ and *My Fitness Pal*™. They are inexpensive apps that help you track total calories, carbs, sugar, exercise…whatever you need to stay focused on your goal. It's up to you to regain your health and maintain your health.

• If you have any health issues, check with your healthcare professional before starting *any* eating plan. One plan does not fit everyone. This is for *your* long term health, not a quick fix.

Step #2: ***Ounces of water — drink more***

• Check with your healthcare professional to make sure you are drinking the correct amount of water for your health.

• If you have no health issues, figure out how much water you need to drink to stay hydrated. There are many articles on the internet that help you determine how much you need to drink every day in relation to your health, amount of exercise you do and the weather conditions in your area

• If the total amount seems overwhelming, start with a glass of water every time you eat something. It makes you aware that you are putting food into your mouth. In turn, it helps to increase your water intake. As a bonus, it makes you feel full and satisfied.

Step #3: ***Out of sight, out of mind***

- Take time to check what you have stored in your refrigerator and your pantry. Become a smart consumer. Check the foods and ingredients that your health care professional or nutritionist have recommended for you and see how many of them you have on hand.

- Read the labels carefully. Just because the front of the package says it's sugar-free, does not mean it has no preservatives or harmful fats, or artificial sugars. If it has ingredients that aren't good for you, and you can't bring yourself to throw it out, give it to a food bank or homeless shelter. You can't eat what you don't see.

- Be wary of what's on television in the evening. Just when you think you've conquered your eating for the day, you may be tempted by those commercials showing delicious, high calorie foods. Close your eyes and take several deep relaxing breaths and remember your "WHY". If that doesn't work and you are still tempted to stroll into the kitchen for a snack, turn off television, read a book or take a walk.

Step #4: ***Don't dwell on mistakes***

- If you eat something you know isn't good for you, don't dwell on it. The world is full of would, could, should moments.

- Mindless eating is something we all do from time to time. The trick is to realize you are doing it, and ...*stop.*

- Think about why you ate it, acknowledge that you ate something that wasn't the best for your health and move on.

- Don't use one bad eating event as an excuse to eat everything in sight.

- Take a deep breath, drink a glass of water, and move forward.

- Ask yourself, "What did I learn from this so I don't do it again?"

Every goal starts with one step. Changing your eating habits may seem overwhelming, but it doesn't need to be.

Make small changes. Be aware of those changes and keep doing them until they become a positive habit. Then move on.

This will be a challenge and it will take effort on your part. But your health is worth the effort. Remember your "WHY".

It's really all about making choices that will help you regain and maintain your health.

- Talk to your health care professional about any health concerns and what type of eating plan is best for you.

- Consult with a nutritionist to develop a plan with the foods that are best for you and your lifestyle.

- I found it was helpful to find a nutritionist who had struggled with her own weight issue. They understand your challenges.

- They will understand what you need to do and help you make the necessary changes.

- Find a nutritionist who is over the age of 40. They understand the changes to your body as you get older, and how difficult it is to just maintain your weight, let alone lose weight. It no longer works to just stop eating desserts.

- Metabolism is like that old clock that sits on the mantel. It gets slower and slower, no matter how much you prod it to move faster.

- Find healthy foods that you like and try new recipes …or old recipes you haven't made in a long time. Find *something* that you like and is good for you.

- Dust off those old diet books. What parts worked for you? Were there recipes that you liked but forgot about?

- Do you have a blender? Make your own smoothie. Save money and empty calories. Be creative. Experiment with different fruits and veggies. There are so many different kinds of "milk" …almond, cashew, unsweetened, sweetened, vanilla, dark chocolate. Find something you like and your stomach tolerates.

- Is there a Farmer's Market in your community? It's a great place to buy seasonal fresh fruits and veggies. You save money, support local farmers and have access to variety of fresh food.

- If you really love that glass of wine with dinner or that bowl of ice cream, don't banish it forever. Be aware of when and how much you are consuming. And don't forget to record it in your food diary. It's amazing how those calories add up.

- Eat fresh whenever possible … seasonal fruits and vegetables are budget-friendly and make for a good variety. I like to make chili in the winter, but don't want to eat it all week. I freeze it in individual containers and pull one out when I don't feel like cooking.

- Enjoy healthy snacks. An apple and a tablespoon of nut butter (cashew or almond are my favorites) is an easy snack that is healthy and tasty.

- Eat healthy meals at home. Then when you go out to eat indulge in a favorite food. Bring half of it home and enjoy it the next day.

Vanessa's Story

A young lady came to my spin class one day in a baggy sweat shirt and sweat pants. She stared at the bike and I could tell she was ready to run out the door. I greeted her and shook her hand. Vanessa had a strong handshake and a look of desperation on her face.

She told me in a quiet voice that she wanted to have a baby, but the doctor said she needed to lose at least 50 pounds to increase her odds of getting pregnant and having a healthy baby. Now, that is a goal! She said she had talked to the nutritionist at the doctor's office and she had suggested that Vanessa start exercising as well as eating the well-balanced diet that had been given to her.

I encouraged Vanessa to start doing the spin class because it would take the stress off her joints while she lost weight, and would give her a good cardio workout. Little did she know just how good the workout would be!

After getting the bike set up for her, she climbed on and held on as if her life depended on it. I told her that she could stop after ten minutes. Everyone else in the class would understand because they had all been there at one time. She shook her head. "I can ride a bike for an hour. No problem." Vanessa lasted 15 minutes.

The important part is that Vanessa came back to class three times a week, increased her time in class every week until she made it through the whole class … and stopped wearing sweats.

More of Vanessa's story later …

Worksheet for this chapter on Healthy Eating

Complete one chart every week. If you didn't complete an item, put a zero. At the end of the week add up your numbers.

Yes   No   Week 1 Date:

☐ ☐ Followed a healthy eating plan this week.

☐ ☐ Ate more fruits and veggies than last week.

☐ ☐ Drank at least 8 glasses of water every day.

☐ ☐ Read labels when grocery shopping before buying.

☐ ☐ Avoided sugar at least one day.

☐ ☐ Ate natural food instead of processed food at least one day.

☐ ☐ Tracked calories and movement

Totals:

Yes   No   Week 2 Date:

☐   ☐   Followed a healthy eating plan this week.

☐   ☐   Ate more fruits and veggies than last week.

☐   ☐   Drank at least 8 glasses of water every day.

☐   ☐   Read labels when grocery shopping before buying.

☐   ☐   Avoided sugar at least 2 days.

☐   ☐   Ate natural food instead of processed food at least 2 days.

☐   ☐   Tracked calories and movement

Totals:

Yes   No   Week 3 Date:

☐   ☐   Followed a healthy eating plan this week.

☐   ☐   Ate more fruits and veggies than last week.

☐   ☐   Drank at least 8 glasses of water every day.

☐   ☐   Read labels when grocery shopping before buying.

☐   ☐   Avoided sugar at least 3 days.

☐   ☐   Ate natural food instead of processed food at least 3 days.

☐   ☐   Tracked calories and movement

Totals:

Yes   No   Week 4 Date:

☐   ☐   Followed a healthy eating plan this week.

☐   ☐   Ate more fruits and veggies than last week.

☐   ☐   Drank at least 8 glasses of water every day.

☐   ☐   Read labels when grocery shopping before buying.

☐   ☐   Avoided sugar at least 4 days.

☐   ☐   Ate natural food instead of processed food at least 4 days.

☐   ☐   Tracked calories and movement

Totals:

Score for each week:

6–7 YES! = You are a super star and well on your way to being healthy after 55

4–5 YES! = You are moving forward and making a positive effort to regain and maintain your health

2–3 YES! = It's time to put more awareness into your choices and accept the challenge of being healthy after 55

0–1 YES! = Evaluate why it is difficult for you to follow these simple guidelines and resolve to do better one day and one week at a time.

NOTE: If you have questions about anything in this book, do your research. Always consult your health care professional before making changes to your diet, medical plan, exercise routine, or anything else that is important to your health. Be informed. Take control. Make the best decision for your health!

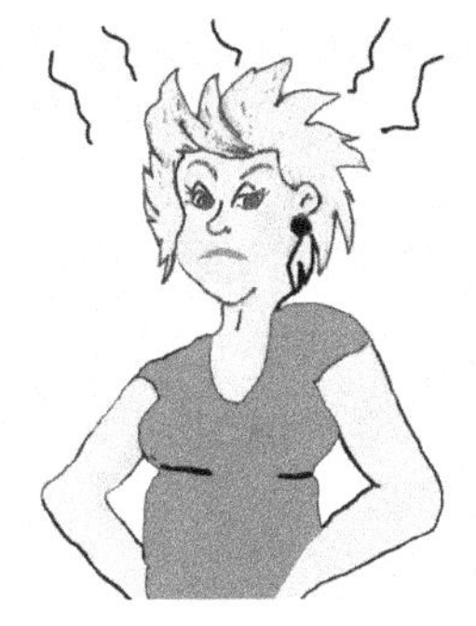

Molly knew this was going to be her biggest challenge.

Every time she had started a new diet, it didn't last two weeks. There was always food at work, and when she worked late, she was too tired to cook, so she would stop at the nearest fast food drive through for dinner.

The first week, she made it through one day eating more fruits.

She managed to drink 6 glasses of water for three days, but had to go to the restroom at work so much, her co-workers asked if she was okay.

Molly read the labels on everything in her pantry, and the shelves were empty by the time she put food with added sugar in a very big box.

She was able to avoid sugar at lunch, but had ice cream every night.

Tracking her movement and food intake was a lost cause. She couldn't remember what she had for lunch and forgot to look at her FitBit at the end of the day.

When she looked at all the 0 on her chart for the week, she knew she had to take a big step …she made an appointment with a nutritionist.

Everything that the nutritionist suggested was reasonable and would work …if she took the time to get prepared for the week.

The second week was still a little bumpy, but by Week 3 she was seeing more YES than NO. Biggest challenge was eliminating sugar even one day a week.

Week 4 was her best week, and when she returned to her nutritionist she had lost 4 pounds and had more energy. She was on her way to regaining her health.

What you learned in this chapter about Healthy Eating.

You learned that diet is more than a four letter word. A healthy eating plan is critical for a long-term healthy lifestyle.

- Follow a healthy eating plan that works for you.

- The amount of water you drink every day is important – count the ounces.

- Out of sight, out of mind. Move the food that is not so healthy to the back of the cupboard or give it away.

- Don't dwell on mistakes that you make along the way. Learn from them and move on.

Chapter #6
Awareness

"Awareness is the greatest agent for change."

Eckhart Tolle

"Did I stop to think about whether this food or activity would help me achieve better health?"

Julie Luedtke

YOU KNOW THAT FOLLOWING THE LATEST DIET trend or thinking about exercising for 30 minutes a day is not going to help you make permanent lifestyle changes. Oh, that it would be true. Think about how much time and money you have spent searching for a plan that would help you lose weight and be healthy with little or no effort.

Every Choice Counts

Awareness of the choices you make every day is more beneficial for long term changes than any new diet trend or exercise plan.

The next time you reach for a candy bar, ask yourself, "Is eating this candy bar going to help me on my journey to better health and wellness?"

If the answer is no, ask yourself a second question, "What will I eat that will help me on my journey to better health?"

Pick up an apple and add some nut butter. Enjoy every bite. You just made the choice to eat something that will help you on your health and wellness journey.

The same question is asked when you think about movement. Ask yourself, "If I sit here and scroll through Facebook for a half hour, will that help me on my journey to health and wellness?"

If the answer is no, then ask the second question. "What activity could I do for 30 minutes that will help me on my wellness journey?"

Go outside, walk around the neighborhood or work in your garden. Bad weather? Turn on some music and dance around the house or clean out a closet.

In the evening when you are watching television, ask yourself, "Is it worth the time and energy to stand up and walk around during a commercial or should I just sit here until it's time to go to bed?"

It takes very little time to stand up and walk around, or go into the dining room and use a solid chair to practice sitting and standing while focused on using your thighs and core.

A small choice with a big reward ... another step toward health and wellness.

As you become more aware of the choices that you make every day, you start to realize that you make choices and aren't aware that you could have done something better, healthier.

It makes sense that the acronym for choices would be **A.W.A.R.E.**

A is for *Aim for healthy choices*
W is for *Watch what you put in your mouth*
A is for *Allow for missteps*
R is for *Reward good choices – no food involved*
E is for *Eat healthy, move more*

Step #1 – *Aim for healthy choices*

This is an important part of your plan for a healthier, happier life.

If you are unsure what a healthy choice might be, do your research. There are many websites and organizations that offer suggestions for healthy food choices. Find one that fits your needs and is easy to use.

There are some foods you already know that are not healthy ... fast food French fries, extra-large milk shake, or eating an entire pizza.

Other choices might not be so obvious.

Should you eat a grilled steak or chicken? The answer is not just the choice of steak or chicken, but what you eat with it. Grilled veggies or French fries?

Consider what you really want to eat, how much of it will satisfy you, and what your ultimate goal is.

Step #2 – *Watch what you put in your mouth*

Sounds simple, but think about today.

What did you eat for breakfast? Lunch? Dinner? Did you snack?

Do you remember everything you ate today?

- Did you eat a whole bag of chips while you watched television when you were only going to have a small bowl?

- Did you eat the leftovers from dinner so you didn't have to store them in the refrigerator?

- Did you devour a bowl of popcorn before going to bed and don't remember eating it?

Be Aware

- Be aware of *what* you put into your mouth

- Be aware of *when* you eat

- Be aware of *how much* you eat.

Check with a registered dietician or your healthcare professional if you have concerns about what you should be eating or if you have physical conditions that need to be addressed. Get the best advice available and *follow it!*

There are many apps to download on your phone to help you track what you are eating and how much you are eating. One of my favorite apps is *Lose It.* You set your goals for weight loss, exercise, calories, water intake, etc. It is user-friendly and gives you gentle reminders to log in.

Start measuring your food

The reality of what a serving size *actually* is and what you *think* it is leads to awareness in a big way.

When I measured my food, I was shocked at how much I was actually eating. No wonder I gained weight. I ate enough for a six foot body-builder.

Step #3 – *Allow for missteps*

This is as important as making the right choices.

Sometimes you really want that ice cream, pizza, or whatever.

Ask yourself those two questions we talked about earlier.

"Is this going to help me on my journey to better health and wellness?" If the answer is no, ask yourself the next question.

"What *will* I eat that will help me on my journey to better health?"

If you still want to eat whatever is lodged in your brain and won't go away, be aware of how much you eat.

Log it on whatever food tracker you use. You will be amazed at how many empty calories you consume. Ignorance may be bliss, but the number on the scale is reality.

Eating something that is not necessarily healthy is a step backward, but limit yourself to a reasonable serving and add enough movement to balance the extra calories consumed.

It is not an ideal thing to do, but it is realistic.

Work on moving forward on your journey to health through realistic, positive choices.

Step #4 – *Reward good choices – no food involved*

Rewards are important. If you have a pet, you already know that. To reinforce good behavior, you give them a treat. They quickly learn what they need to do to get that treat.

Humans are similar. Rewards reinforce good behavior. The difference is that we need to give ourselves rewards that don't involve food.

It would be wonderful if you could reward yourself with a treat every time you made a healthy choice. I would be the first person in line for that reward!

Use your imagination. When you make a healthy choice, give yourself a pat on the back. Look in the mirror, smile and say, "I deserve to be healthy. Well done!"

Positive reinforcement works whether we are speaking to someone else or our own image in the mirror.

As we talked about in the first book, make **JOY** a priority every day. Just One Yes is a great way to reward your wise choices. Think about what you did that was positive. Say YES and give yourself a hug.

Remember the "*WHY*" when you have a choice to make. *WHY* your health is important to you. *Why* your wellness is a priority.

Set a large reward when you accomplish a big goal. Maybe your reward is a special manicure or a new workout shirt or tickets to a movie you've wanted to see. When you reach your goal, enjoy the reward. You've earned it.

The bigger the goal, the bigger the reward

Write the goal and the reward on a piece of paper.

Put it where you will see it every day.

Positive reinforcement.

Step #5 – *Eat healthy, move more*

This sums up what this book and chapter are all about. Healthy eating and more movement.

It's about awareness of what you are doing and what you need to do to regain and maintain your health.

This doesn't have to be difficult.

Instead of sitting for an hour and watching television, stand up and walk around the room. Practice your balance.

Instead of eating a bowl of ice cream in the evening, eat a piece of fruit or have a cup of tea.

Make small changes and become aware of your choices. Make a positive difference in the quality of your health.

More about Vanessa...

Vanessa took that first step by trying a spin class and following the healthy eating plan suggested by her nutritionist.

She became aware of her eating habits and stopped her frequent visits to fast food restaurants for lunch or dinner. She made her own meals and followed a simple eating plan. She tracked her food intake every day.

Vanessa gradually increased her movement from spin class twice a week to three times a week. Then she slowly added walking and strength training.

In five months, Vanessa had accomplished her goal of losing 50 pounds and was determined to lose more weight.

She bought cycling shorts and started to wear sleeveless workout shirts. She asked for a training plan to go from walking to running.

A couple of months later, Vanessa asked if she could join me for a 5k (3.1 miles) race. We did the race together. I don't know who was more thrilled when we crossed the finish line. She gave me a big hug and said she had not only lost another ten pounds, but she was pregnant!

One step at a time...

Worksheet for this chapter on Awareness

Every day for a week write down one time you were aware of making a choice to move forward on your health and wellness journey.

	Awareness	Healthy Choice
Day 1		
Day 2		
Day 3		
Day 4		
Day 5		
Day 6		
Day 7		

At the end of the week, think about the choices you had and the ones where you chose to eat or move in a healthy manner.

If you made more than 5 healthy choices, do something positive for yourself…reinforce the positive behavior.

Remember **JOY** Just One Yes for yourself!

Molly thought this would be easy. She was eating healthier food and drinking more water.

She set a goal for the week. She hadn't gotten a pedicure in months and she wanted to wear a new pair of sandals she had purchased for the summer. Seemed like a doable goal. She could make five positive choices. No problem.

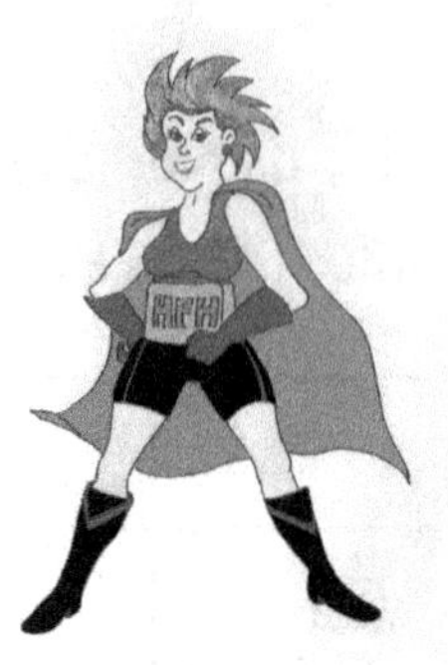

Day 1 – Molly ate a piece of birthday cake at the office without even thinking about it … until her plate was cleaned off.

She still had six days to reach her goal.

Day 2 – Molly had a choice to go for a walk after work or go out for a drink and dinner with a friend. She chose dinner with the friend. And ate fried chicken instead of a salad.

She had five days to reach her goal.

Day 3 – Molly chose a healthy salad at lunch instead of a hearty sandwich. Finally put a mark in the Awareness column.

Day 4 – Molly made her own smoothie for breakfast and took it to work. Another mark in the Awareness column. Three more to reach her reward.

Day 5 – Molly reached for a bag of chips when she made a quick trip to the grocery store. She stopped, read the label and slowly put it back on the shelf. She really wanted that pedicure.

Day 6 – Molly had the choice of going back to sleep or going for a walk. She thought about how her goal and what a difference being aware of her choices made to what she did. She got out of bed and went for a walk.

Day 7 – Molly looked at the paper she had taped to her bathroom mirror. She really wanted that pedicure. She looked at her feet and the new sandals sitting her closet. She had to be vigilant today.

Molly was aware of everything she put in her mouth during the day. She took a walk instead of a nap in the afternoon.

She had one more choice to make. A glass of wine with dinner or ice tea.

Molly chose the ice tea. Hot Flash Holly appeared on the table in front of her and gave her a high five! She did it. Awareness plays a huge role in making healthy choices.

What you learned in this chapter about Awareness.

You learned that awareness is an important part of developing a healthy lifestyle.

- Be aware of choices you make every day

- For every choice you make that helps you move forward, give yourself a non-food reward.

- Don't dwell on mistakes that you may make along the way, learn from them and move on

- Eat healthy foods and increase your movement to reach your health and wellness goals.

NOTE: If you have questions about anything in this book, do your research. Always consult your health care professional before making changes to your diet, medical plan, exercise routine, or anything else that is important to your health. Be informed. Take control. Make the best decision for your health!

Chapter #7
Choices

"We are a product of the choices we make, not the circumstances that we face."

Roger Crawford

"Life is just one choice after another. Choose to be healthy!"

Julie Luedtke

AWARENESS AND CHOICES GO TOGETHER LIKE SPRING and flowers.

Think about the choices you make *today* to start the journey to regain your health.

Pause for a moment and think about it. Choices are made without even thinking about it. Many times we are overwhelmed by circumstances in our lives. How many times in the past have you made choices for someone else's happiness rather than your own? How many times did you put the needs of your partner, child, or work before your own need to be healthy? Now you know why it is so important to *choose* to be healthy.

If you are over the age of 55, you've survived many predicaments where circumstances were beyond your control. But you still needed to make choices and those choices affected how you moved forward with your life.

Perhaps now you are overweight and have difficulty walking up a flight of stairs. You could live for another 30 or more years. Is this how you want to spend the rest of your life? Wishing you could do more, but unable to make the choice to be healthy?

Your *choices* now affect how you live your life for years to come. Will it be your best life or merely survival?

It makes sense that the acronym is **C.H.O.I.C.E.S.**

C is for *Choose to be healthy*

H is for *Help someone else be healthy (accountability)*

O is for *Opt for healthy foods*

I is for *Increase your movement*

C is for *Come clean – get rid of processed foods*

E is for *Enjoy how you feel*

S is for *Smile in the mirror at the healthy person looking back*

Step #1 – *Choose to be healthy*

If that sounds like an awesome task, it can be. But if you take it one step at a time, it won't be so overwhelming … and the rewards are worth the effort.

Think about some ways you might choose to be healthy. You will find many of the same choices in this book as in the first book. Yes, I am repeating these choices because they are so important that you need to hear them more than once.

Think about *why* you want to be healthy.

It's important to really think about this … something other than just to lose 20 pounds. Is it to attend your grandchild's wedding in 15 years? Do you want to take the stairs at work rather than the elevator? You want to avoid the diabetes the doctor said would develop if you don't start eating right and moving?

What is really important to *you*? Not the person in the ad who wants you to buy their product. Not your neighbor who runs marathons. Not your friend who follows every trendy diet on the market. What is important to *you*. When you make the right choices, your life is more enjoyable, and you increase your health and wellness.

Go back to the first chapter and really think about your "why". Why is health and wellness important to you?

Now, write it down and post it on your refrigerator and the mirror in the bathroom. Add a photo of your grandchildren or family members. Look at that reason every time you need to make a decision that will affect your health.

Don't feel like taking a walk today? Look at your "why", lace up those shoes and go outside.

A bag of chips is so much easier to grab than slicing an apple. Think about your "why" and take two minutes to prepare the apple, sit down and enjoy it.

Do you see where we are going with this?

We talked about awareness in the last chapter. Now that you are aware of making choices every day, it is time to make conscious choices that will help you regain and maintain your health.

Step #2 – *Help someone else be healthy (accountability)*

One way to increase your chance of success in making healthy choices is to help someone else be healthier, too. It could be a spouse, good friend, co-worker or neighbor. Someone you share the good choices with and someone who understands when your choices aren't quite so good and will encourage you to keep moving forward.

Consider this person your accountability buddy. You both want to be healthier and make decisions that will increase your health and wellness.

You don't have to share every detail of your journey, but when you know you are going to have to tell a friend that you just don't feel like meeting to take a walk, you will probably put on your shoes and take a walk.

One accountability buddy that will really hold your feet to the fire is one of your children. They love the fact that they hold you accountable. My daughter relishes being able to give me the "look" when I reach for ice cream instead of fruit. She says it's payback for all the times I gave her that look when she was about to do something she knew she shouldn't do when she was growing up. Be careful what you ask for. My neighbor was much more sympathetic to my errors in judgment.

Maybe you want to keep this new focus on your health to yourself. There is nothing wrong with that if you feel you are able to maintain the focus on changing your lifestyle for years to come.

You will be amazed at the support you will receive if you reach out to someone and ask for their support. You will be helping them as well as you both travel the winding road to lasting health and wellness.

Step #3 – *Opt for healthy foods*

This is obvious, I know. You've heard me say this many times already in this book as well as the first one. Healthy foods are important to your overall health and wellness.

If you haven't done so already, this is also a good time to talk to your healthcare professional or a certified dietician about any health issues you have and what foods are best to eat and what you should avoid. The answers may surprise you.

I thought I was eating foods that were good for me and would help me lose a few pounds. When I proudly presented my food diary to a nutritionist, she looked at it and then at me and shook her head. "You aren't eating enough quality calories to sustain the activities you are doing. No wonder you have no energy and aren't losing the inches." That was an *aha* moment for me. I always thought less calories and more exercise was a good thing. Not necessarily.

That's when I followed her advice. I finally lost a few pounds and had more energy. I not only ate more quality foods, but I also increased the *quality* of my exercise rather than the quantity.

Ultimately, it really is a matter of choices. It may seem easier to put a frozen dinner in the microwave rather than prepare a homemade meal, but it's not that difficult to make a wise choice.

Purchase a blend of salad greens, add a serving of tuna, some tomatoes, and a healthy dressing and you have a healthy meal.

The key is to have healthy alternatives in your kitchen.

If you open your pantry door and the first thing you see is a bag of chips and a box of cookies, guess what you will eat without even thinking about it. This is the voice of experience speaking.

Step #4 – *Increase your movement*

We've talked about this before. You know how important movement is to your health, but are you aware of all the positive things that happen to your mind, body and emotions when you start moving more?

Recent studies have shown that movement helps your mood be more positive, increase your ability to sleep better and rev up your metabolism.

Movement is crucial to helping you regain and maintain your health. Movement is anything from standing up at work and walking around the office to going for a hike on a Saturday morning. It could be as simple as walking around the block or working in your yard. It might be walking around the whole grocery store before you start to put anything in your cart or washing your windows.

Your mind and body are connected. The choices you make with your mind will affect how your body works. And the reverse is also true. The choices you make to move your body will affect how efficiently your mind works.

The choices you make with your body affect how your mind reacts to stress, joy, depression and peace.

These choices seem small, but they are a great way to start if you've been inactive for some time.

Note: If you have been inactive, have any health limitations or concerns, please see a health care professional before doing any activity. The goal is to regain your health, not hurt yourself.

Step #5 – *Come clean – get rid of processed foods*

One of the biggest complaints I've heard about eating healthy foods instead of processed food is the cost.

It seems expensive to buy fresh fruit and veggies or grass-fed beef, rather than the pre-packaged or fast food dinner.

Think about it. The fast food dinner has more bad fats, calories and preservatives than the fresh food. What are you saving if you have to go to the doctor to treat your high blood pressure, need insulin for your diabetes, or joint replacement due to your excess weight?

There are plenty of ways to save money while eating healthy. Buy frozen fruit and veggies that haven't been processed. Buy chicken, fish or meat when it's on sale and freeze it in individual portions. Visit your local farmer's market.

Again, it's all about taking one step at a time. Your health and wellness are worth every step.

Step #6 – *Enjoy how you feel*

Think about how you feel when you walk just a little further each day.

Think about your feeling of accomplishment when you eat a salad for dinner rather than a pizza.

Think about how good you feel when you pass up the ice cream and purchase frozen veggies instead.

You've spent most of your adult life helping other people around you feel good about themselves. Not it's time to feel good about the choices you are making for yourself.

Be proud of what you are doing. The journey takes time. Every step forward is a reward.

Step #7 – *Smile in the mirror at the healthy person looking back*

Sometimes this is the most difficult thing to do. Usually when we look in the mirror, we see everything wrong with the image looking back at us. Wrinkles, grey hair, etc.

Take the time to smile at your reflection. You are making healthy choices, you are regaining your health. *You are worthy of wellness.*

Worksheet for this chapter on Choices

Every day for a week write down just one time you had to make a choice to move forward on your health and wellness journey or do nothing.

Sunday ____

Monday ____

Tuesday ____

Wednesday ____

Thursday ____

Friday ____

Saturday ____

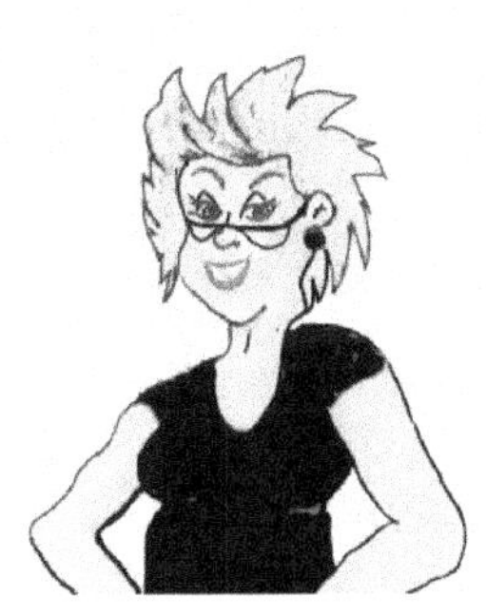

Molly was feeling pretty good about herself as she became more aware of her decision.

Hot Flash Holly added positive feedback as Molly moved forward toward health and wellness.

Molly thought after doing the worksheet on awareness, the worksheet on making healthy decisions would be easy.

Life got in the way.

Just as Molly was feeling positive, she had to make a quick trip from Los Angeles to New York on Sunday afternoon.

She tossed some protein bars in her purse, wore her walking shoes and was sure she could make healthy choices during the three days she was away from home.

Sunday passed in a blur and by the time she looked at her worksheet, she realized she hadn't made any healthy choices. She couldn't remember what she ate or did, but it wasn't healthy.

Hot Flash Holly sat on her shoulder as Molly looked in the mirror on Monday morning. "I just need to make one choice to day that will help me toward my health and wellness goal," Molly muttered.

"I have faith in you," Hot Flash answered. "You can do this."

Molly made the decision to walk five blocks to work instead of asking for the company limo. Hot Flash Holly gave her a thumbs up and sat on Molly's shoulder as they walked to work.

The rest of the week was a challenge, but every day Molly was conscious of making at least one decision that would move her toward health and wellness.

It wasn't as difficult as she thought it would be as long as she practiced awareness.

What you learned in this chapter on Choices.

You learned that choices are an important part of developing a healthy lifestyle.

- Be aware of choices you make every day

- For every choice you make that helps you move forward, give yourself a non-food reward

- Eat healthy and move more to reach your health and wellness goals.

- Come clean – banish foods that delay your progress

- Enjoy how you feel when you make wise choices

NOTE: If you have questions about anything in this book, do your research. Always consult your health care professional before making changes to your diet, medical plan, exercise routine, or anything else that is important to your health. Be informed. Take control. Make the best decision for your health!

Chapter #8
Restart

"In two decades I've lost a total of 789 pounds. I should be hanging from a charm bracelet."

Erma Bombeck

"I can't count the number of times I've restarted, but I will continue to pause, restart and move forward on my wellness journey."

Julie Luedtke

WE MIGHT LAUGH AT THE QUOTE BY ERMA BOMBECK, but we all relate to the challenge of starting a new eating plan with high hopes, maybe join the local gym, lose a few pounds, and then.. old habits and patterns of eating and sitting in front of the television or sleeping an extra 30 minutes resurface and we give up.

How many times throughout your adult life have you tried a new diet or exercise routine, maybe lost some weight, felt better and then you made a misstep. You gave up and returned to old habits. Then you had to pull out the old, larger sized clothes that you always kept …just in case.

We've All Been There!

How do I know this has happened to you? Because it has happened to me more times than I care to remember!

And that is one of the reasons why I decided to write this series of books. I've experienced it all and learned many lessons through the years. It was time to give back to help women who have struggled to regain and maintain their health after 55.

After talking to so many women in the same stage of life and listening to their experiences, I knew how important a healthy lifestyle is for all women over 55.

This book is about making *permanent* lifestyle changes. Your health and wellness depend on it.

None of us are perfect. We all make choices that are not so healthy. Do you really want to go out to eat with friends and not have a glass of wine or a special meal? You need to have joy in your life and do some things that may not be the healthiest choice, but they give you joy.

This chapter is about realizing you aren't perfect and you will make some unhealthy choices. That is when it is crucial to take a deep breath and step back onto the path of health and wellness.

This is a journey that will have rocks, pot holes and weeds as you wind your way along the journey to reach your goal of regaining and maintaining your health. That doesn't mean you throw your hands in the air and give up when you make an unhealthy choice.

Of course, the only acronym that makes sense would be **R.E.S.T.A.R.T.**

R is for *Regrets are banished*
E is for *Engage in positive self-talk*
S is for *See how far you've come*
T is for *Take your worksheet out – why did you start?*
A is for *Allow yourself to reevaluate how to proceed*
R is for *Return to your worksheets and regain momentum*
T is for *Take control of your health*

Step #1 *– Regrets are banished*

Health and wellness are a lifelong journey.

It took years to get unhealthy. It will take time to regain your health.

If you continually look in the rear view mirror, and think about what you could have done or should have done, you will never see the great opportunities in front of you.

Think about it. Can you do anything about the decisions you made yesterday, last week or last year? Not really.

Do you think about how "bad" you were and ignore making better choices? Banish those thoughts.

Learn from those decisions. Plan your day so you make healthy choices.

Remember your "why". The choice is yours.

Do you want a healthy, vibrant life for the next 20, 30 or 40 years?

Do you want to sit in a chair as an observer and not a participant in the lives of your friends, children and grandchildren?

Do you want to travel with friends or stay home because you are unable to keep up with them?

Choices you make every day will decide what choices you are able to make in the future.

That's the reality of restarting the journey for your health and wellness. Not just once or twice, but every day.

Every choice is a building block toward your goal to regain and maintain a healthy life.

Banish the regrets and continue to move forward.

Step #2 – *Engage in positive self-talk*

We talk to ourselves all the time.

What we say is important to our body as well as our mind. You cannot disconnect the mind from the body, or the body from the mind. Whether you like it or not, they work together.

Think about what you have said to yourself in just the last hour.

"I'm too old to do that."

"It costs too much money to eat healthy."

"I don't have the energy to walk around the block. It won't do any good anyhow. I'm fat."

"No one else cares about my health. Why should I care?"

Does any of that sound like something you've said to yourself?

Now think about how you will change those words into something positive.

"Other women are doing this and they are older than I am. I will do this for myself!"

"I will figure out a way to eat healthy and save money. I just need to be creative."

"I may be slow, but I will walk around the block. My health and wellness journey has to start somewhere."

"This is all about me. It's time to be selfish!"

Positive self-talk makes a difference not only in your attitude, but also the choices that you make.

The next time you start to have a negative thought about yourself and your health, *stop*. Think about how you will turn that thought into a positive action. Then do it.

Ester's Story...

A few years ago, when I was running local 5k races, there was a 72-year-young lady who would walk the first few blocks with her walker. She always had it decorated for the season. In the spring she had flowers all over her walker and at least one flower tucked behind her ear. Santa races were the most fun. I'd see her with twinkling lights on her walker and a Santa hat tilted on her silver hair. She would wear crazy sunglasses and always be laughing and smiling.

I stopped to walk with her one day and told her she was my role model. She laughed and shook her head. "I'm not a role model. I have Parkinson's and have to keep moving to stay alive. I just choose to have fun while I do it."

She has since passed away, but her memory and her positive spirit live on for me.

Step #3 – *Look at how far you have come*

This is one time to look back over the past week or month, or whenever you started your health and wellness journey.

Were you able to walk around the block or walk a mile when you started on this journey?

Were you able to walk up a flight of stairs instead of taking the elevator?

Did you make conscious choices to eat healthier or do things that would increase your wellness?

Did you complete worksheets from prior chapters or from the first book?

Think about the positive steps you have taken to regain and maintain your healthy lifestyle.

Remember **JOY** and give yourself a hug. You've earned it!

Step #4 – *Take out your first worksheet – remember why you started this journey*

This is an important step if you have wandered off your path to health and wellness.

It is hard to wrap your brain around the goal of health. It's not like a goal of saving $20. That's a tangible goal. Health is a more difficult goal to set. It's hard to know when you've achieved it. It's all about motivation.

When you start to waiver, you make poor choices. It's amazing that you work for such a long time to correct bad habits and yet they rear their ugly heads when you least expect it.

Take your worksheet out from the first chapter and read your "WHY". *Why* did you start this journey in the beginning? What was important to you then? Is it still important or have you changed your priorities?

These are questions that only you can answer. It's important to think about what motivates you to be healthy.

Take some time to think about your answers before you move forward. Think about what has changed in your life. Update your "WHY" and post it on the refrigerator or bathroom mirror. Look at it every day.

Take a deep breath and move forward … one step at a time.

It's Time to Re-Examine

If your "why" is not meaningful, you will find every excuse to step back onto your journey of health and wellness.

Look at other worksheets you have completed. Look at your goals, the steps you've accomplished, the goals you want to reset and what you want to change.

Think about what motivates you and make that a priority.

Think about Ester. Her motivation was to stay alive. Walking was her priority to reach that goal.

Step #5 – *Allow yourself to reevaluate how to proceed*

None of this process or these goals is written in stone.

Maybe your initial "WHY" was to lose 10 pounds before your annual physical checkup. You went to the doctor and were told that your weight is okay, but you need to move more.

Great. Now you need to decide if you are going to listen to the advice of your doctor, or continue with your original plan just to eat healthier.

Are you going to reevaluate what you need to do to add more movement to your daily routine or ignore it? Just when you thought you had a plan … it changes.

The choice is yours. How are you going to proceed? What goals are you going to change?

Perhaps there have been life changes since you started this journey. What seemed like an easy, manageable goal a month ago has changed into a huge challenge.

There is nothing wrong with reevaluating your goals. The important thing is to keep moving forward … in spite of the rocks and boulders that have appeared on your life's path. You sit down and give up, or you find a way around the boulders to reach the other side.

Revise your goals and move forward.

Step #6 – *Return to your original worksheets and regain momentum*

If you printed your worksheets and completed them, it's a great idea to return to them. Read them and think about where you started. Print new ones and restart where you need the motivation.

Your circumstances may have changed, but what about your goals? Have you accomplished any or all of them? Are they still relevant?

What new goals will you set or what goals can you go back to and reset?

Remember, it's a journey for the rest of your life. There may be detours, but the objective is to get back on the road to health and wellness.

I hear you right now. "Sure, it's easy for you. You've been active and healthy all your life. You don't know what it's like to have to start all over."

You are so wrong! Yes, I've been active and healthy most of my life, but when menopause knocked on the door, I welcomed the excuse to stop working out and ate everything except the wallpaper.

A visit to the doctor was my whack on the head. I had gained 20 pounds, my cholesterol was out of control, triglycerides were horrible, and my blood pressure was inching toward unhealthy.

A friend wanted me to go with her on a fund-raising weekend bike ride, but I wasn't sure I could do it.

That was the jolt I needed. It was time to reset my priorities. I created the worksheets that you are using right now. I worked hard to change the bad habits I had adopted. I set my goal of joining my friend on the bike ride.

I made some bad choices at first, but started to see positive results. Chocolate continues to be a nemesis for me, but it's a work in progress.

Sharing my story with you is important. You need to know that you are not alone in this journey. So many women have shared their stories with me and continue to struggle just as we all do. You need to remember this journey is worth the time and effort.

Step #7 – *Take control of your health*

And that takes us to this important step.

After reevaluating your original goals, once again think about your "WHY". Look at your worksheets. Think about how far you've come. It's time to take control of your health and wellness.

I've said it before and I will say it many times …

This is a journey of a lifetime.

The phrase that life is a marathon, not a sprint, may be overused, but it's so true. Your objective is to be healthy and live a vibrant life as long as possible.

If you are 55, you could live another 30 or 40 years. How do you want to live those years? Some things regarding your health are out of your control, but there are so many things that you control with the choices you make.

When I went to the doctor's office for my annual checkup, I was struck by the number of older adults who were probably younger than I am but were walking with walkers or in wheel chairs. The most shocking thing was to see several of them finishing a cigarette before going into the doctor's office! It is so sad to see their choice was cigarettes rather than health.

Are you going to let smoking or a fast food restaurant control your health?

Are you going to listen to your overweight friend who says it's a waste of time to walk around the block?

No one has control over your health except for you. It's your life, your body, your health. *It's your choice.*

Worksheet for this chapter on Restarting

Every day for a week, write down one time you thought about giving up and what you did to restart your health and wellness journey.

Sunday ____

Monday ____

Tuesday ____

Wednesday ____

Thursday ____

Friday ____

Saturday ____

Small steps lead to big changes!

Remember your "WHY".

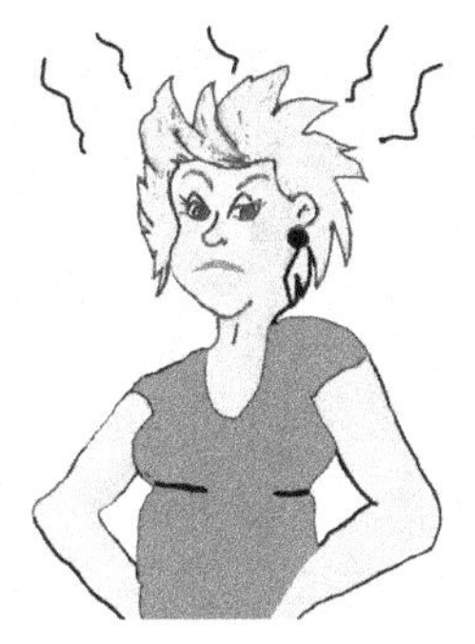

Molly was going to ignore the worksheet for this week. She thought she had a good routine going and was feeling very positive about her progress.

Until she went out with friends on a Saturday night, had too much wine, stayed out late, and decided to stay in bed Sunday morning instead of going for a walk.

By three o'clock in the afternoon, she had eaten a container of ice cream and was drinking wine instead of water.

She stumbled into the bathroom.

Hot Flash Holly was standing on the counter, her hands on her hips. "How can you make so many bad decisions in one day?" she demanded.

Molly shrugged. "Does anyone really care what I do? Is it going to make any difference if I make healthy choices or not?"

Hot Flash shook her head. "Think about your WHY."

Molly paused for a moment and thought about that. If she didn't take care of herself, who would do it? Her children had their own lives to live. She didn't want them to have to take care of her because she had ignored her health until it was too late. She was looking forward to playing with her grandchildren someday.

She took out the worksheet and wrote down what she had done, why she thought about giving up, and her reason for starting in the first place.

Hot Flash Holly landed on her shoulder and smiled. "One day at a time, Molly. One step at a time."

What you learned in this chapter about Restarting.

You learned that sometimes it is important to restart your journey toward a healthy lifestyle.

- Banish the regrets as you restart.

- Change negative self-talk into positive talk.

- Don't dwell on mistakes that you may make along the way. Learn from them and move on.

- Look at your worksheets and remember why you started your healthy journey.

- Reevaluate where you are, where you want to end up, and how you want to proceed.

- Take control of your health. No one else will do it for you.

NOTE: If you have questions about anything in this book, do your research. Always consult your health care professional before making changes to your diet, medical plan, exercise routine, or anything else that is important to your health. Be informed. Take control. Make the best decision for your health!

Chapter #9
Lifestyle Changes

"Your life does not get better by chance. It gets better by change."

Jim Rohn

"The first step toward change is awareness. The second step is acceptance."

Nathaniel Branden

"Make positive changes to regain your health."

Julie Luedtke

THESE QUOTES SUM UP THE WHOLE CHAPTER ON change.

It's All About Increments

The first step is mental. By now you have an awareness of what you need to do to make healthy choices.

It may seem overwhelming at times to make all these changes in your eating and movement choices, but it's your choice to look at it as depressing and too much work or …as a challenge and fun.

The second step is acceptance. Accept that you need to make changes to regain and maintain your health. It won't happen if you just wish for it. There is no magic involved here.

One step at a time.

Of course the acronym for this chapter is **C.H.A.N.G.E**

C is for *Choose what you eat and how you move*
H is for *Have faith in your ability to create new healthy habits*
A is for *Awareness of bad habits replaced with healthy habits*
N is for *Nothing worth having is easy*
G is for *Get moving*
E is for *Energy – use it wisely*

Step #1 – *Choose what you eat and how you move*

We've talked about choices in every chapter. That's because we make choices all the time and need to be aware of what we are doing.

Think about your current day.

You had a choice to get out of your comfy bed and get your day started or stay in bed.

You had to make a choice of what to wear for the day, what to eat for breakfast.

Some of these choices you make without even thinking about it. It's a habit.

Start thinking about the choices you make regarding what you eat. Do you plan healthy meals and snacks?

Do you make deliberate choices to move during the day?

Do you take the elevator to your office on the second floor without even thinking about walking up the steps? Could you walk up one flight of steps?

Small choices lead to big changes.

Step #2 – *Have faith in your ability to create new healthy habits*

Self-doubt is like a worm in your brain. It starts small and then winds its way into all your thoughts and decisions.

We already discussed how we talk to ourselves all the time. It's time to talk positively to your inner self-doubt.

The next time you hear that little gremlin in your head say, "You are too old to do that," banish the thought.

Instead say to yourself, "I am never too old to regain my health. It's worth it to me to make healthy choices. I am worth it!"

Step #3 – *Awareness of replacing bad habits with healthy habits*

Awareness is the key to replacing bad habits. Those habits don't go away, they just hibernate until you aren't looking and then poke a hole in your good intentions.

I wish I could count the times I thought I had replaced the bad habit of eating something sweet after lunch or dinner. I would have a piece of fruit or drink a big glass of water. Maybe it worked for a few weeks, and then, just when I thought I had conquered that particular bad habit, someone at work would have a birthday and bring in doughnuts. Of course they would place one on my desk.

The darn doughnut just dared me to ignore the chocolate icing. Yes, I took a big bite and then thought about how hard I had worked to replace the bad habit with a healthy habit. I shocked myself by spitting it out and throwing the doughnut in the garbage. Amazing.

That doesn't mean the bad habit was gone forever. It went back into hibernation mode waiting for another chance to win the habit battle.

This little story just illustrates how difficult it might be to change bad habits into healthy ones.

Not all habits are as difficult to change as my battle with sweets.

I like to work out, so putting on my workout clothes and heading outside or to the gym is an easy decision to make.

We all have our gremlins that want to challenge our choices to lead a healthy lifestyle.

The important thing is to be aware of easy choices for you and reinforce them. Then be aware of the difficult choices and try to prepare for them. Awarenss is key.

Step #4 – *Nothing worth having is easy*

We all know this. Think about your life. The things that mean the most to you are the things you had to work hard to achieve.

The steps on your journey to health and wellness will be difficult. Many of those steps will seem like you are climbing a mountain ... and maybe you are. The view from the top will be worth the effort.

Take a moment to close your eyes and imagine yourself at the beach. You love coming to the beach and walking along the water, picking up shells along the way.

Now, think about walking along the beach and you aren't sure you will walk a block. Bending over to collect shells and carry them would be too much effort.

Is that how you want to live the rest of your life? Think of the things that gave you so much pleasure and now are too much of an effort.

Step #5 – *Get moving*

No choice here. Just move.

No excuses.

Movement is crucial for your health and wellness. Start with small steps.

It is important to check with your health care professional to make sure you are able to do the things you want to accomplish. This is all about improving your health, not getting injured.

Put on comfortable shoes and walk around your neighborhood.

Park your car a little farther away from the store when you go grocery shopping.

Walk up a flight of stairs instead of taking the elevator.

Walk around the office every 20 or 30 minutes … even if it's just to the restroom.

When you go to the park and watch your kids or grandchildren play, walk around instead of sitting down.

Step #6 – *Energy – use it wisely*

Energy is positive or negative.

"Your positive action combined with positive thinking results in success."
Shiv Khera

Think about that. If you've gotten this far in this book you are already thinking about positive changes you will make in your life.

Use the worksheets and take the steps necessary to regain and maintain your health.

Small steps lead to big changes.

Worksheet for this chapter on Healthy Lifestyle Changes

What are the top five things you want to change in your life?

1. ____

2. ____

3. ____

4. ____

5. ____

What are five steps you will take to change one of the priorities above?

1. ____

2. ____

3. ____

4. ____

5. ____

For the next five weeks, each week choose one thing from the list above that you want to change and focus on the steps to create that change for a week. Each week add another change you want to make.

Week 1 ____

Week 2 ____

Week 3 ____

Week 4 ____

Week 5 ____

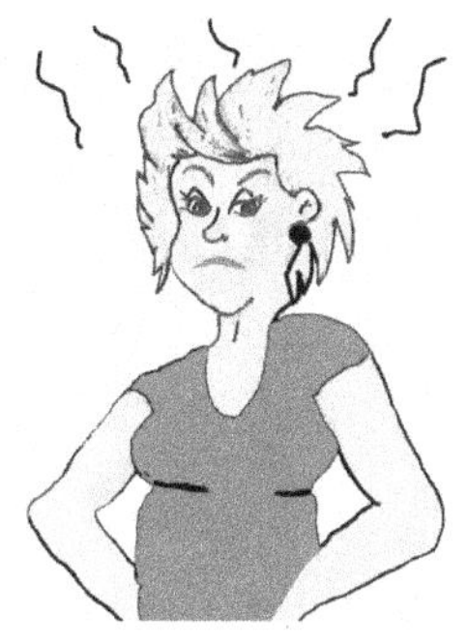

Molly knew this worksheet would be difficult to accomplish, but she thought she would give it a try.

She wrote down the top five things she wanted to change.

She looked at the list and decided for the first week she would focus on reducing the amount of sugar she ate. She wouldn't try to eliminate it completely the first week, just try to reduce the amount she ate.

Her five steps included using her app to record everything she ate and how much sugar she was consuming.

Another step was to make more meals from scratch to eliminate added sugar.

The most difficult step was eliminating her glass or two of wine every evening. She hadn't realized how much sugar she was consuming.

That first week was difficult, but Hot Flash Holly kept encouraging her to keep moving forward.

The second week she started to meditate to reduce the stress in her life. That proved as much of a challenge as reducing the sugar she was eating. It wasn't easy to meditate when her mind was moving like a snow globe, but she kept trying.

The third week she started taking a yoga class after work. She scheduled it on her calendar and made it through three classes that week. Hot Flash Holly was there to help her and remind her of why she was going to yoga class instead of her favorite bar after work.

The fourth week she bought a cook book with healthy recipes and made healthy dinners every evening.

The fifth week she started a gratitude journal. It was time to be glad she could make the changes she was doing.

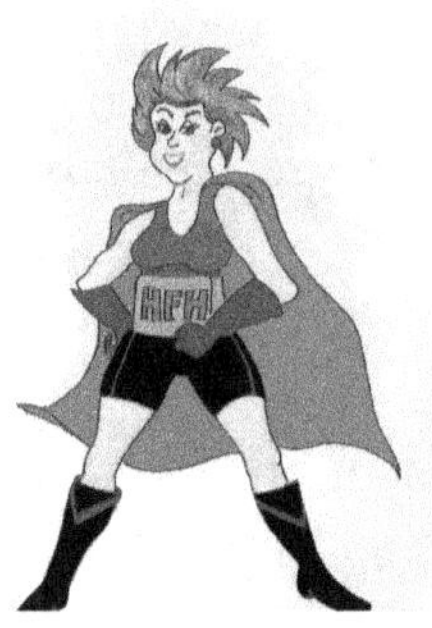

What you learned in this chapter about Healthy Lifestyle Changes.

You learned that choices are an important part of changing your lifestyle to be healthier.

- Choose what you eat and how much you move.

- Have faith in your ability to create healthy habits to replace the unhealthy habits.

- It's worth the effort to regain your health.

- Think of creative ways to get moving. No more excuses.

- Use your energy wisely as you move forward.

NOTE: If you have questions about anything in this book, do your research. Always consult your health care professional before making changes to your diet, medical plan, exercise routine, or anything else that is important to your health. Be informed. Take control. Make the best decision for your health!

Chapter #10
What's Next

"Small steps lead to big changes. Are you ready to take small steps to accomplish your big change?"

Julie Luedtke

IT'S TIME TO PUT ALL THIS INFORMATION TOGETHER to create healthy habits and make smart choices.

The Time Is NOW

We discussed movement and the importance of taking the steps necessary to strengthen balance.

We talked about food choices and creating awareness regarding what we eat and how we move.

We even discussed restarting when we fall back into old unhealthy habits.

And we stressed the importance of small steps that lead to big changes.

It makes sense that the acronym for the final chapter in this book would be **N.E.X.T.**

N is for *Now is the time*
E is for *End negative thoughts*
X is for *X-tend your vision*
T is for *Take another step forward*

Step #1 – *Now is the time*

Now is the time. Not tomorrow. Not next week or next month.

Procrastination rears its ugly head when we least expect it. Acknowledge it, take a deep breath and move beyond it.

Take it from the voice of experience. This happens to me more times than I care to admit. Sometimes I give in for a few days or a week, but then I write down my "why" and set new goals. I put this in the "present" tense because it is an on-going battle that needs to be addressed daily.

The challenge never stops, but the goal you set is worth the effort.

Now is the time to eat healthy foods and move more.

Make choices to regain and maintain your health.

Step #2 – ***End negative thoughts***

End those negative thoughts that swirl around in your head.

It's never too late to start the journey to a healthy life.

Remember your "why" and take positive steps to make your goal a reality. You know it won't be easy. You know it will take effort.

One of the most important decisions you make is to take control of your health. Regain and maintain. Those are the thoughts that should knock down negative barriers.

The journey will have twists and turns … even a few boulders along the way.

The view from the top as you regain your health and vitality is worth every step you had to take to accomplish your goal.

Step #3 – ***X-tend your vision***

Your goal to regain your health as you change your habits and bring awareness to your choices is on two levels.

Immediate – one change at a time, think about what you are doing right now. *Today.*

Long term – extend your vision and your goal.

Are you planning a trip and you want to be able to walk all day and experience as many new sights and sounds as possible?

Are you looking forward to playing with your grandchildren? Do you want to get down on the floor to play with them and then stand up without help?

When is your next check-up with your health care professional? Do you want to hear positive results from blood work? Blood pressure numbers better than the last visit?

Look forward and increase your awareness. It's up to you to make the decisions and set goals that will regain and maintain your health.

Step #4 – *Take another step forward*

Set reasonable goals, write them down, and when you reach them, give yourself a hug. You've earned it.

Remember the "JOY". Just One Yes! For you. You are worth it.

Worksheet for this chapter on What's Next

It's time to set short term and long term goals as you move toward a healthier lifestyle.

Write down three short term goals you want to accomplish. One might be to walk 20 minutes every day. Another might be to drink more water every day. Put dates on the worksheet when you want to accomplish your goals. Make the goals and the dates realistic.

Think about two long term goals you want to achieve. Maybe you want to lose 15 pounds or take a trip with friends to another country. Put a date on these goals, too, but make sure they are reasonable.

Short term goal ____

Short term goal ____

Short term goal ____

Long term goal ____

____

Long term goal ____

____

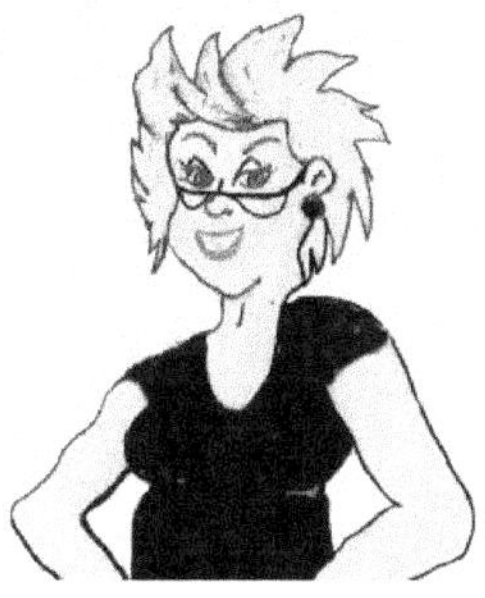 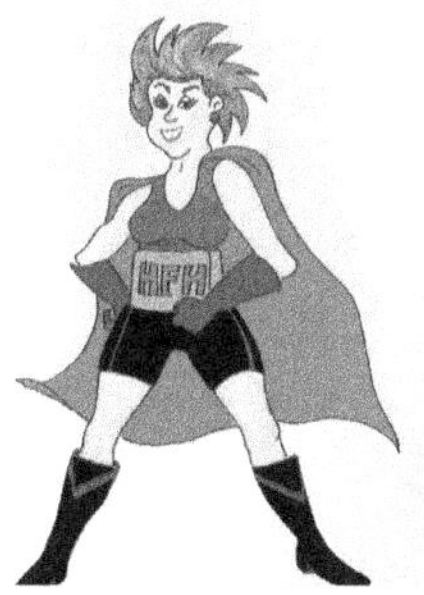

Molly thought about this worksheet for an hour or more. She would write down a goal, then change it. Three goals seemed overwhelming.

Hot Flash Holly flew around her head and landed on her shoulder. "Molly, Molly, Molly. You are over thinking this. Start with something simple. How about drinking eight glass of water every day for one month and track it. Short and simple. Just do it."

Molly thought about that for a moment and then nodded her head. "Good idea. Short and simple."

She chose two more short and simple goals. One was to walk 20 minutes every day for one month. Another was to continue her yoga class but do it three times a week instead of two.

Long term goals took a little more time. She really wanted to eliminate the 15 pounds of fat that had settled around her waist, but wasn't sure how she was going to accomplish it. She set a long term goal of one pound a week for 15 weeks. That was a reasonable goal.

Her second long term goal was to join a group of friends on a trip to England. They had planned it one night at dinner and she thought about joining them, but had decided it was too expensive and she would be gone from work too many days. She decided to make it a priority, save her money and save her vacation days. Work would still be there when she returned.

Hot Flash Holly clapped her hands and cheered for Molly. It wouldn't be easy, but each goal was achieveable.

> ## What you learned in this chapter about What's Next.
>
> You learned that awareness is an important part of developing a healthy lifestyle.
>
> - Now is the time to move forward with healthy choices.
>
> - Banish negative thoughts.
>
> - Don't dwell on mistakes that you make along the way. Learn from them and move on.
>
> - Think about your "why" and how important your health is to you and your loved ones.

NOTE: If you have questions about anything in this book, do your research. Always consult your health care professional before making changes to your diet, medical plan, exercise routine, or anything else that is important to your health. Be informed. Take control. Make the best decision for your health!

Chart Your Progress

Use this chart to set your goals for each day/week. Be realistic and start with just one attainable goal and then adjust your goals as you reach each one.

Have a calendar that you will see every day when you wake up and before you go to bed.

Write on the calendar what you want to accomplish that day. When you accomplish it for the day, put a sticker or check mark in that square. Try to accomplish more goals each week.

Week 1 – Set 2 goals – keep it simple

Week 2 – Set 2 additional goals

Week 3 – Set 2 additional goals

Week 4 – Review past 3 weeks. Look at what you *have* accomplished and how far you've come. If you haven't reached your goals, restart and renew your determination to regain your health.

Week 5 and beyond – Set additional goals, review how far you've come and keep moving forward.

About the Author

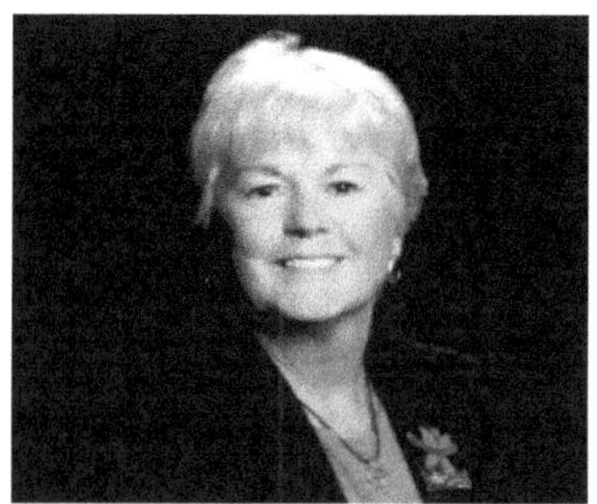

JULIE LUEDTKE is a certified personal trainer and certified to train older adults. She lives in Phoenix, Arizona where she teaches exercise classes for older adults. She lives what she teaches. At 74, she still does half marathons and other events that challenge her. Julie loves educating and inspiring adults to live life to the fullest … no matter what their birth certificate says.

Learn more about Julie at amazon.com/author/business

See videos for more detailed instructions presented here on her Facebook page Healthy After 55.

Learn more about how Julie will help you regain and maintain your health at HealthyAfter55.com

One Last Thing...

If you enjoyed this book or found it useful I'd be very grateful if you'd post a short review on Amazon. Your support really does make a difference. I read all the reviews personally so I receive your feedback to make the next book even better.

Thanks again for your support!

NOTE: Nothing in this book should be considered medical advice. Always consult a doctor before making any changes to your diet, medical plan, exercise routine or anything else that is important to your health. Be informed and make the best decision for your health!